Advanced
EXERCISES IN DIAGNOSTIC RADIOLOGY

13

COMPUTED TOMOGRAPHY OF THE BODY

HELEN C. REDMAN, M.D.

Associate Chief of Radiology,
Mount Zion Hospital, San Francisco;
Clinical Associate Professor of Radiology,
Stanford University and University of
California, San Francisco

ALLAN E. FISCH, M.D.

Assistant Chief of Radiology,
Department of Radiology,
Mount Zion Hospital, San Francisco;
Clinical Instructor of Radiology,
University of California, San Francisco

W. B. SAUNDERS COMPANY • PHILADELPHIA • LONDON • TORONTO

W. B. Saunders Company: West Washington Square
Philadelphia, PA 19105

1 St. Anne's Road
Eastbourne, East Sussex BN21 3UN, England

1 Goldthorne Avenue
Toronto, Ontario M8Z 5T9, Canada

COMPUTED TOMOGRAPHY OF THE BODY

Advanced Exercises in Diagnostic Radiology — 13   ISBN   0-7216-7492-5

Last digit is the print number: 9   8   7   6   5   4   3   2

ACKNOWLEDGEMENTS

Many people have helped to make this book possible. Our colleagues in the Radiology Department at Mount Zion Hospital have been tolerant of our preoccupation and have kept us informed about interesting scans as they have occurred. Drs. Alan J. Davidson, Barton Lane, Jerome Jacobson and Phillip Brodey have been especially helpful in this regard.

Our CT technician Nafisa Patel has consistently produced excellent scans, cajoling reluctant patients into breath holding. She has also made copies of the examinations for the photographer with the areas of interest displayed to the best advantage. Her backup technicians Marvin Hom, Patty McGrogan, Albert Hom and Gerry Toriumi also have not let us down.

Special thanks must go to the many radiologists in the San Francisco Bay area who gave us cases to fill the gaps in our experience. This book would have been much longer in preparation without their generous assistance. Dr. Jerry Parker provided cases 2–4, 2–10, 2–16, 3–7, 4–5 and 7–4. Dr. Jay Mall lent us 2–5, 2–15, 3–3, 6–4, 8–4 and 8–6. Dr. Jan Kaiser sent us cases 3–8, 4–2, 4–8, 4–13 and 5–10. Dr. Brian Salman donated cases 2–7, 2–15, 3–3, 6–4, 8–4 and 8–6. The teaching file from which all these cases were drawn is a fascinating encyclopedia of CT body scanning pathology. Mr. M. L. in case 4–6 was supplied by Dr. Robert Koch, and Dr. Klaus Dehlinger provided case 8–3. Drs. James McCort and Robert Filpi lent us cases 3–12, 3–13 and 5–5. Cases 2–6, 3–4, 3–11, 5–3, 5–6, 6–1 and 7–14 were supplied by Drs. Ronald Castellino, Barbara Carroll and George Harell from the Department of Radiology at Stanford University Medical Center. Last, but certainly not least, Dr. Harry Genant provided the four bone cases, 9–6, 9–7, 9–8 and 9–9 from his experience at University of California, San Francisco Medical Center. Since we do almost no bone CTs, this was very valuable assistance. Dr. Paul Guttman provided the ultrasound for case 3–14.

Mrs. Cheryl Candia deserves great credit for her patient typing and retyping of the manuscript through its many versions. Completion of the book probably pleases her as much as it pleases us.

CONTENTS

INTRODUCTION

Computerized tomography (CT) became a reality for the brain about five years ago and has revolutionized neuroradiology. The fact that a CT brain scan can replace cerebral angiography and pneumoencephalography as a diagnostic tool and even provide information that was inaccessible in the past has made the application of CT to other areas of the body exceedingly attractive.

Computerized tomographic scanners have been more difficult to develop for the body than for the head. The brain is conveniently encased in bone and can be held motionless while the shapes of abdominal organs vary widely; these organs have no hard boundaries to facilitate computer program writing and require air gap scanning techniques. Respiratory, peristaltic and vascular motion cannot be completely stopped. These considerations have resulted in the development of several generations of CT scanners with rapid scanning capabilities, and more sophisticated computers and computer programs. Fortunately, more attention has also been given to patient comfort and care. For the moment the pace of technological advance has slowed and more clinical experience is being obtained. The place of CT body scanning in the diagnostic armamentarium can now be evaluated.

This book is intended to give the reader an overview of CT anatomy of the body with its many variations, to demonstrate pathological conditions and, most important, to illustrate situations in which CT body scanning can play a primary or backup role in diagnosis and management of the patient's condition.

The patients whose cases are discussed and illustrated in this book are real and the diagnoses are correct as far as is known; however, not every case is pathologically proven. Clinical histories and the progression of diagnostic studies have been modified when necessary so that situations are illustrated in which CT has a significant clinical application. We have tried to demonstrate the CT findings in the more common diseases that might be encountered in clinical practice. We wish to emphasize that ultrasound examination of the abdomen and pelvis often provides as much or more information than CT scanning and should be performed first in patients with suspected abdominal and pelvic problems since it is simpler, more versatile and does not use ionizing radiation. If ultrasound is technically unsatisfactory or inconclusive, then CT can be considered. Ultrasound may seem very fallible in this book, but use of cases in which ultrasound failed is necessary to justify a CT examination in specific clinical situations. So our apologies to ultrasonographers. There are, of course, several situations in which ultrasound is of limited use, such as evaluation of the urinary bladder, bone and any air-containing structure. In these situations, CT should generally be used first.

This book should be approached in an orderly fashion, since the cases tend to be more complex at the end of each chapter and understanding of each chapter presupposes knowledge gained from the earlier chapters. We suggest you sit down with a good cross sectional anatomy book at your elbow and go through this volume from start to finish. If later you wish to refresh your mind about a specific area, reading that section will probably suffice.

CHAPTER
1

TECHNIQUE

CT body scanning is a new art and so techniques will vary from institution to institution and from one type of CT body scanner to another. There are some technical points common to all units that you should know and several principles of CT scanning that you need to understand in order to properly utilize and interpret the examinations.

SCANNING TIME

Because the older CT body scanners have scanning times of 2.5 to 5 minutes, the patient must breathe quietly throughout the study. This causes some motion artifact and, in general, obscures small structures since the gentle respiratory excursion of upper abdominal organs is at least 1.0 to 1.5 cm. These scans lack the sharp definition of those done on more advanced equipment, but it must be emphasized that much useful information can be obtained from studies done on the slow scanners.

The newer scanners take between 1 and 30 seconds to complete a body scan. Almost any conscious patient can hold his breath repetitively for 3 to 5 seconds but repetitive breath holding is much harder even for the healthy adult during scans requiring 18 to 30 seconds. Children and extremely ill adults have a difficult time cooperating at even the shortest scanning times. Scans in the primary area of interest should be done first to ensure maximum patient cooperation. Hyperventilation before each section can help with breath holding as can the breathing of oxygen. It should be remembered that one gasping respiration will cause more serious artifacts than several small ones, so if a patient cannot hold his breath for the entire duration of a scan, it is generally better to let him breathe quietly.

VIEWING SCANS

The convention in body scanning is to view the scan as if you are looking from the patient's feet and so, on a supine scan, the patient's right will be on your left as you view the film or display screen. This is the orientation of the standard radiograph and should not be confusing. The prone scan will be reversed on the display screen using this viewing convention, but, in this book, to decrease confusion, the patient's right will always be on your left as you look at the CT scans. Scanning units can generally be programmed to display all scans in a standard orientation if desired.

POSITIONING

Most units are capable of scanning patients in the supine, prone and decubitus positions. The patient beds are generally designed for supine scanning, so the patient is most comfortable in this position and can cooperate most fully. Prone and decubitus scanning should be reserved for situations in which they are necessary.

Positioning of patients for specific examinations varies from institution to institution but cannot be as routine as in head scanning, since patients vary greatly in size and shape. Because each body scan should be tailored to the individual problem, positioning must be decided upon at the time of the examination. Review of other radiographs, ultrasounds or radionuclide scans is important when positioning the patient. A radiograph with appropriate markers can be taken to locate the area of interest when needed and some institutions use ultrasound for assistance in positioning. In general, however, after an initial section in the approximate area of concern, subsequent scans can be appropriately performed.

NUMBER OF SCANS IN AN EXAMINATION

Most scanners have a scan thickness of about 1 cm; therefore, scanning at closer intervals in the body is seldom indicated. In fact, since respiratory excursions vary organ position and since the patient cannot hold his breath in an identical position for each scan, there is rarely a reason for scanning at less than 2 cm intervals. Abdominal surveys for adenopathy or to determine the extent of a known mass can be carried out at 3 or 4 cm intervals with more frequent scans added in areas of specific interest.

The number of sections to be obtained will also vary with the questions to be answered and with body size. As few sections as possible should be done to decrease radiation to the patient. Close attention to the study as it is in progress is necessary to achieve this goal.

USE OF CONTRAST MEDIA

Contrast media are frequently used in CT body scanning. Dilute water soluble contrast material is given to opacify the stomach and the small bowel. This is done to delineate the bowel from adjacent structures. Nonopacified bowel loops can be confused with masses or enlarged lymph nodes. A very dilute solution of contrast medium is used to avoid obscuring small structures. All barium-based contrast materials are too dense for this purpose. Intravenous contrast material is used to identify blood vessels, to locate the ureters and to enhance attenuation differences between normal and abnormal tissues. The volume and timing of such usage will depend on the goals of the specific examination. Oral and intravenous gallbladder contrast agents are sometimes used for studies of the biliary system. Dilute water soluble contrast medium or air may be given by rectum if it is necessary to identify or distend the large bowel. Other markers such as tampons placed in the vagina are occasionally indicated.

ARTIFACTS

Motion of any sort causes artifacts on CT scans. Fast scanners have decreased the artifacts caused by respiratory motion, but peristalsis, vascular pulsation and actual patient movement remain problems. When peristalsis is likely, glucagon or an "atropine-like" drug can be given to temporarily diminish peristalsis. Sedation may diminish patient motion when reassurance about the procedure does not produce full cooperation. Vascular motion is unavoidable with current equipment, though in the future, scanners used for thoracic scanning are likely to be gated with the EKG to diminish cardiac pulsation. At present all thoracic scanning has some motion-induced image degradation.

Other causes of artifacts are retained barium, metallic prostheses and surgical clips. In general, any very high density object is likely to cause artifacts when included in the plane of the scan. Another source of artifact is the computer program itself. Extremity scans, for example, frequently have artifacts caused by the unusual distribution of air and bone. The computer is not programmed to accept this distribution and usually produces a spray or circular artifact as a result. Some of the more common artifacts are illustrated.

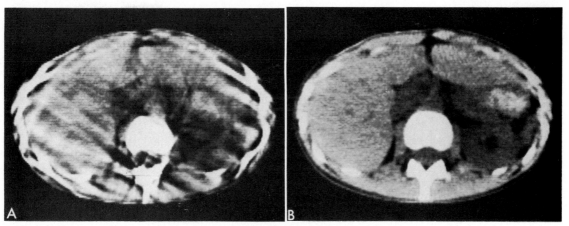

FIGURE 1–1a, b

Scans *a* and *b* from a study done on a young woman with metastatic osteogenic sarcoma who was afraid of the scanning unit. She feared that she would be "sawed in two" and could not hold still. Scan *a* has many linear streaks caused by motion and respiration. Only the spine can be identified and it is distorted by the motion. Scan *b* done at the same level, after sedation, shows good detail of the liver, left kidney and pancreatic tail. The patient is very thin, so the fat planes that help in distinguishing the various organs are poorly developed.

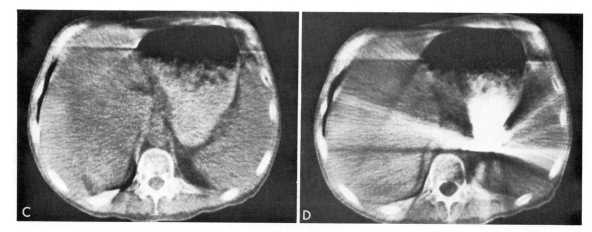

FIGURE 1–1c, d

Scans *c* and *d* demonstrate two more problems. Scan *c* shows the liver, an enlarged spleen and the stomach, which contains air and dilute contrast material mixed with food. A slight streak artifact runs through the liver from the stomach, possibly caused by some gastric peristalsis. The whiteness around the streak near the stomach is a typical artifact generated by an internal interface of air and soft tissue. It is an inconstant artifact more common with some scanners than with others but should be recognized as a computer-induced artifact.

Scan *d* is at the same level. It was done after more concentrated contrast material had been given. The glucagon used to cause temporary cessation of peristalsis has worn off and the dense contrast material is shooting off extensive artifacts. Again the gastric contents are seen floating in the contrast medium solution.

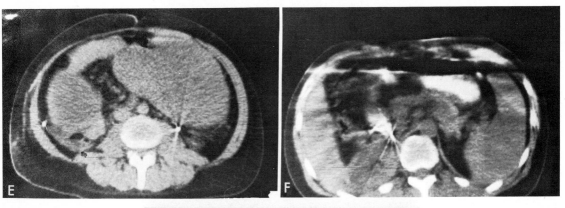

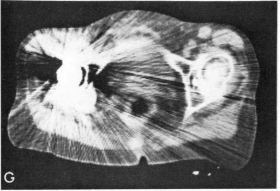

FIGURE 1–1e, f, g

Motion is not a necessary component of all artifacts, though it makes most worse. Scans *e*, *f*, and *g* illustrate this. Scans *e* and *f* were done on a young man with a recurrent liposarcoma. For scan *e*, the first section performed, the patient held completely still. Even so there are radiating streaks from the metallic surgical clips to the left of the spine and near the right lateral abdominal wall. Later in the study, the patient was tired and took one breath during a scan at the level of the pancreas. The coarse, linear artifact is caused by the breath. A metallic clip to the right of the spine is giving off larger streaks and cannot be separated from the duodenum, which contains contrast medium that is too concentrated.

Scan *g* is on another patient who has a metallic total hip prosthesis. She held still for this section, but the computer program generated these extensive artifacts. The computer program simply cannot assimilate the attenuation readings received from such a large metal object. It produces massive streak artifacts, as well as erroneous findings adjacent to the prosthesis. It may be possible to place such a patient in the gantry obliquely to exclude the metallic object from the scan. Computer programs to eliminate this type of artifact may also be developed. With current technology, however, these artifacts are difficult to avoid unless the metallic object can be removed from the plane of the section.

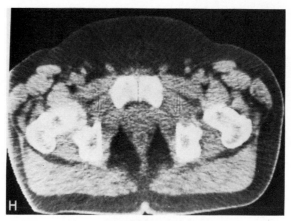

FIGURE 1–1h

Scan *h* has a subtle artifact that does not really reduce the diagnostic information in this patient. There are bilateral lines, which run ventrally from the pubic bones near the acetabula. This type of artifact is inconstant but tends to occur more during studies of the pelvis or extremities. It is circular in configuration with some scanners and can be serious enough to diminish diagnostic information. Figures 5–4 *e* and *f* are good examples of this problem.

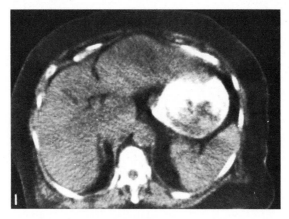

FIGURE 1–1i

This patient was being evaluated for a left upper quadrant mass. Oral contrast medium has been given and this section at 2 cm below the xyphoid tip shows the stomach with a large filling defect. A gastric carcinoma could look like this, but in this patient the mass is lunch. Patients do not need to fast for most body scanning but in some situations fasting may be necessary. Repeat scan in this patient when the stomach was empty was normal except for the large left liver lobe.

The artifacts that have been illustrated are generally easily recognized. While most cannot be totally eliminated, their incidence can be decreased by careful attention to the problem at hand. Patients can be reassured or sedated. Peristalsis can be quieted. Metallic objects can often be removed from the plane of the section by judicious angling of the gantry or oblique placement of the patient. As computer programs are improved, these problems diminish. There are patients who are impossible to scan and artifacts that are unavoidable, but these should be few.

Scanners have many individual idiosyncrasies that the operator should learn in order to get the best possible study from the machine. The most important point in CT body scanning technique is that each procedure must be tailored to the problem at hand and to the patient with that problem. There is no such thing as a completely routine CT body scan.

GLOSSARY OF CT TERMS

ARTIFACT — A portion of the CT image that does not represent anything really present in the patient. Artifacts degrade the diagnostic quality of the image. The two main sources of artifacts are patient motion and errors in the data collecting or processing system.

ATTENUATION — As x-rays pass through the various tissues of the body, a portion of the beam is absorbed or scattered. This loss of x-rays from the x-ray beam is called attenuation and differs in various tissues. The CT image is produced by measuring the attenuation of the x-ray beam in many very small areas, integrating the information and projecting the resulting data in picture form on a television screen. Graded shades of gray are assigned to different degrees of attenuation.

ATTENUATION NUMBER — A scale of numbers ranging from −500 to +500 is used on most CT scanners. These numbers have an assigned mathematical relationship to the linear attenuation coefficient, itself a mathematical representation of attenuation. The "attenuation" of air is −500, whereas the "attenuation" of water is at the midpoint of the scale or 0. +500 is the "attenuation" of bone. These numbers may be referred to as CT numbers or Hounsfield numbers.

CONTRAST — The property of an image that is determined by the degree of difference between the whitest and blackest parts of the image. This is measured as change in optical density. An image of high contrast will have a marked change in optical density between its darkest and lightest areas.

CONTRAST MEDIA — Contrast agents, materials or media are often referred to as "contrast" and include any substance used to alter the inherent ability of tissues to attenuate x-rays. This effect should not be confused with the property of the image that is called contrast. Contrast materials may be placed directly into a hollow viscus or body cavity or may be administered intravascularly or orally to reach the target organ through the blood stream.

The contrast media used in radiography include positive and negative agents. Positive contrast agents are those that are of greater x-ray attenuating ability than water and include iodinated water soluble organic compounds, iodinated oils and barium salts. Barium sulfate, the most commonly used contrast medium in gastrointestinal radiology, is not used in CT scanning because it is very dense and is a consistent source of artifacts. Water soluble tri-iodobenzoic acid derivatives are widely used in general radiology and in CT scanning. The most commonly used compounds are diatrizoates or iothalamates prepared either as sodium or meglumine salts. These compounds are used intravenously and increase the attenuation of blood and vascular tissues. They are excreted by the kidneys and therefore increase the attenuation of the renal excretory system. Vascular organs such as liver and spleen and some pathologic processes will also have an increased attenuation after administration of these contrast materials.

Dilute solutions of these compounds can be used to opacify the hollow viscera. They are widely used in the stomach and small bowel and may be given by enema to opacify the large bowel or by catheter to opacify the bladder.

A group of compounds are excreted by the liver into the biliary tract and these may be used in CT scanning to opacify the biliary tract and gallbladder. Oral agents, most commonly iopanoic acid, and intravenous compounds such as iodipamide meglumine are available.

Iodinated oils have a wide variety of uses in radiology but are of little use in CT scanning because they persist in the body for a long time, have a very high attenuation and can cause artifacts. In this volume, iodinated poppy seed oil, the contrast agent used in lymphography, will be encountered in a few patients who had already had lymphography.

Negative contrast media are those of lesser attenuating ability than water. These are gases, most commonly room air or carbon dioxide. It is obvious that the use of such a material is confined to the body cavities and hollow viscera. Gases can be introduced directly into the viscus by catheter or needle or may be introduced in the interstices of a fibrous pad such as a vaginal tampon. Powders that release carbon dioxide are available for use in the upper gastrointestinal tract. Air provides "natural" contrast material in the lungs and gastrointestinal tract.

CT SCANNER COMPONENTS

Gantry — The portion of the CT scanner that houses the x-ray source and detectors and provides a mechanism to move these around the patient. The gantry generally surrounds and supports the bed on which the patient is examined.

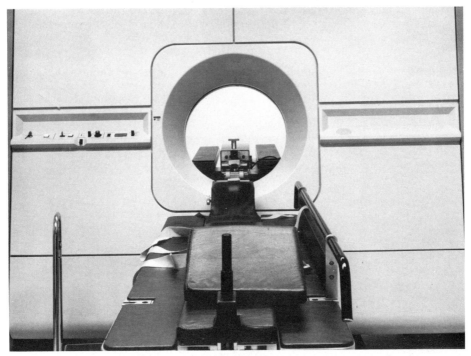

FIGURE 1–2

This is a typical appearance of a CT gantry. The area of the body to be examined is placed in the ring-like aperture. The patient examining table has been totally withdrawn from the scanning gantry in this illustration. The apparatus seen through the gantry aperture engages the examining table when it is in place. The patient lies on the raised central portion of the bed. This slides into the scanning aperture during the examination. The head holder is designed for supine scanning and can cause difficulties in other positions. The side rails are used during patient transport.

On the gantry are controls for gantry angulation and bed position. There is also an intercom, which is used to communicate with the patient during scanning.

Collimator—A device for controlling the thickness of the x-ray beam. In most commercially available CT scanners, the collimator may be varied to produce x-ray beams of different thicknesses. The thinner the examining beam, the thinner the final CT section. In the abdomen, the collimator is generally set to produce a beam of 10 to 13 mm. Moderate changes in collimation cannot be detected visually in the abdomen and at present there is little reason to vary it.

Detector—A device that is sensitive to ionizing radiation. The detectors in a CT scanner produce a quantitative electrical impulse when the x-rays that have traversed the patient reach them. This electrical signal is transmitted to the computer for processing. Various detector types and arrays are available.

Computer—The computer is used to store data collected during the scanning process and to perform the calculations needed to produce the final pictorial image. The computer also stores the programs that control the functioning of the system and the various data processing and manipulating programs.

Console—The control panel of the scanner that allows the operator to contact the computer, to initiate or stop the scanning process, to manipulate the image parameters and to view the image. Console components vary from scanner to scanner.

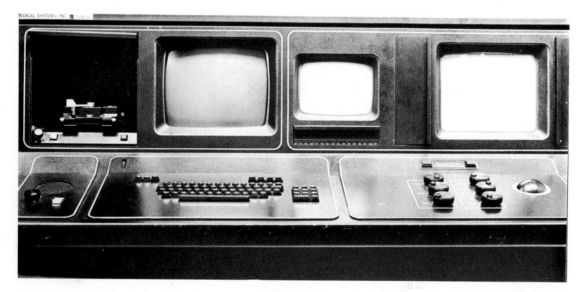

FIGURE 1–3

A typical CT console is illustrated. This particular console includes, from left to right, a camera and an intercom, a teletype keyboard and a video screen for communication with the computer and two monitor video screens with dials for adjustment of window and mean. The hemisphere seen at the extreme right allows manipulation of a cursor "dot" for the measure mode and for linear measurements.

GRAY SCALE — The pictorial display is produced in a specific range of gray tones which are assigned attenuation values. The gray scale extends from black to white. Black generally represents −500 and white +500, though this can be altered. Only a small portion of the 1000 unit scale is used for most examinations. In the usual display, air (−500) is black, while dense bone and metallic prostheses (+500) are white. The intervening soft tissues are presented as shades of gray. The number of shades used will vary from scanner to scanner. A color scale is also possible.

IMAGE RECONSTRUCTION — The production of a spatial image based on the x-ray attenuation data obtained during a scan. This is done by the mathematical process called "convolution" or "filtered back projection." In this process, a series of attenuation profiles obtained at different angles of view of the subject are mathematically back-projected onto the spatial matrix to produce the final image.

IMAGE STORAGE — Most systems have a variety of image data storage methods, generally including magnetic tape or disc. The image data may be stored or studied as a paper printout of the attenuation data. The pictorial image may be photographed from a console monitor for ready viewing and interpretation.

MATRIX — A mathematical grid that divides the scan into many small individual picture elements. This grid is the framework for the computer-reconstructed image obtained in CT scanning but it is never visualized. The "fineness" of the matrix refers to the number of picture elements in the matrix and is expressed by giving the number of picture elements along each axis of the grid, for example, 180 × 180.

MEASURE MODE — All modern CT scanners have a means of measuring the attenuation number in a given small area which is designated by the examiner. The number is generally seen on the display screen.

PARTIAL VOLUME — The CT image not only has length and width but also has depth. This depth varies in different instruments but is generally about 1 cm in body scanning. If a structure occupies the total depth of an image, its attenuation will be accurately portrayed. If it occupies only a portion of that depth, the attenuation shown will be an average of the object's attenuation and those of other structures inferior or superior to it in the section.

PATIENT POSITION — The orientation of the subject in space. In all CT scanners now in use, the patient bed is horizontal, parallel to the floor. The position of the patient is described in relation to the patient bed.

Supine — The dorsal surface of the patient is against the patient bed.

Prone — The ventral surface of the patient is against the patient bed.

Lateral Decubitus — The stated side of the patient is against the scanning bed.
   Supine CT body scans are generally viewed in the same orientation as conventional radiographs with the patient's right side on the left side of the image. Some scanners also present prone scans in this fashion while others do not. The orientation in lateral decubitus scans will depend on which side of the patient is against the patient bed. This position is often difficult for patients to maintain.

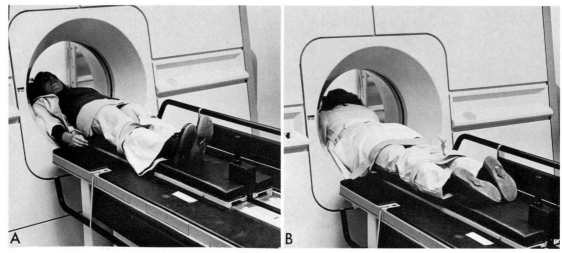

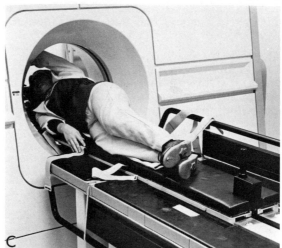

FIGURE 1–4a, b, c

A technologist demonstrating the supine, prone, and lateral decubitus positions.

PIXEL — An individual two-dimensional picture element. These units are usually about 1 mm × 1 mm. The picture element also has a depth determined by the thickness of the x-ray beam being used. For this reason, an individual picture element is sometimes thought of as having volume and is called a voxel.

RESOLUTION — Resolution is a measure of the ability of an imaging system to distinguish and discriminate between small structures. In CT scanning, the maximum theoretical resolution of a scanner is determined by the pixel size of the system. In practice, however, the degree of resolution is larger than the pixel size.

TOMOGRAM — An image of a body slice in a specific plane. In CT scanning, the slices are perpendicular to the long axis of the body. The tomogram is like a slice pulled from a loaf of bread.

WINDOW MEAN OR MEAN — The point along the −500 to +500 scale where the image window is centered. This point determines, along with the window width, which attenuation numbers and therefore which structures will be displayed on the display screen. This can also be varied by the examiner. This may also be referred to as "window level."

WINDOW WIDTH — The range of CT numbers encompassed in a single gray tone on the visual display. This may be varied by the examiner to demonstrate areas of interest to the best advantage. The wider the window, the more CT numbers per gray tone and the lower the contrast. Though the image may seem better, generally information is decreased. In some systems window width is simply called "window."

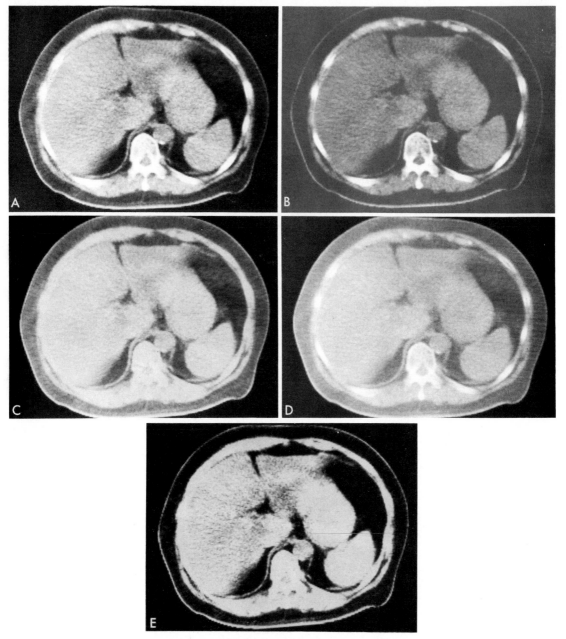

FIGURE 1–5a, b, c, d, e

A single body section has been reproduced after various adjustments of window mean and window width. In scan *a* the two factors have been set to produce the best evaluation of soft tissue structures in the abdomen. It is still possible to identify some bony detail. In scan *b* the mean has been raised and the bony detail is improved, while soft tissue detail is decreased. It is possible to raise the mean further and evaluate only the bones. Scan *c* has a mean too low for soft tissue detail.

Scans *d* and *e* show the effects of window width manipulation. In *d* the window has been made too wide. This produces an image of low contrast with an obvious loss of soft tissue detail. Scan *e* shows the effect of a very narrow window. The image has high contrast but little detail. Images like this are sometimes useful in the display of marked differences in tissue x-ray attenuation.

CT SCANNING OF THE LIVER

Computerized tomography has significant advantages in the evaluation of the liver because the hepatic parenchyma is directly visualized. Only ultrasound and isotopic studies can also demonstrate hepatic parenchyma. In other radiographic techniques such as angiography, the liver substance is not visualized, but changes within it are implied by the abnormalities seen in adjacent structures.

All of these techniques have individual advantages and the choice of procedure should depend on the specific problem. In some patients, the techniques should be used in an appropriate sequence as required; in others, several tests will be needed from the start to obtain a diagnosis.

Hepatic CT scanning is best employed to examine mass lesions. Differences in attenuation characteristics of the mass and of the substance of normal liver make detection possible. Sometimes the attenuation characteristics of the mass and its interface with the liver can be used to determine the specific nature of the abnormality. More often, only location, configuration and number of lesions are determined. Extension of a mass beyond the hepatic capsule can also be demonstrated.

Diffuse changes in CT attenuation may be seen in certain metabolic abnormalities of the liver such as hemochromatosis or fatty infiltration. These processes are generally incidental findings during examinations done for other reasons.

Intravenous contrast material plays an important role in CT evaluation of the liver. When contrast medium is given there is a generalized increase in attenuation of the liver substance. When this occurs a mass that previously had the same density as the liver will generally stand out from the normal liver substance, since most lesions do not take up contrast material to the same extent as the liver. A lesion that is seen prior to administration of contrast medium is usually seen better after the contrast medium is given, and the nature of its interface with the liver is more clearly demonstrated. Blood vessels and very vascular masses may increase their attenuation to equal or exceed that of the liver after contrast medium. For this reason, the liver should almost always be examined before and after intravenous contrast material is given to avoid missing any lesions.

The larger bile ducts and blood vessels are seen on CT scans. Generally, they radiate out from the porta hepatis and, while a tubular structure may be demonstrated, more often the shape is ovoid or round. Bile ducts and portal veins both have a lower attenuation than the liver parenchyma. Attenuation of the portal veins is enhanced by the usual intravenous contrast media; agents specific for the biliary system must be used to opacify selectively the gallbladder and bile ducts.

It is important to realize that while CT scans of the liver can often provide the answers to a diagnostic dilemma, other modalities are also available that can do the same thing. It is important to approach each patient individually and choose the procedure most likely to provide the needed information with the least cost and hazard to the patient. Therefore, at the present time, radionuclide scans should generally be used first when mass lesions are considered and ultrasound when an obstructed biliary system is the problem. CT scanning should be reserved for those patients in whom the answer is not obtained by the first study and for unusual situations in which no other modality could provide the desired information, such as detection of a fatty liver.

MRS. B. R.

Mrs. B. R., a 46 year old woman, is referred for CT scanning to assist in staging of a histiocytic lymphoma recently discovered in a right axillary node. She had an oral cholecystogram earlier in the day because of a history of fatty food intolerance. The CT scans are performed at 2 cm intervals through the liver.

The initial section is obtained at 1 cm above the xyphoid. Dilute oral contrast medium has been given and is seen in the gastric fundus. Are there any abnormalities? Identify all the structures present.

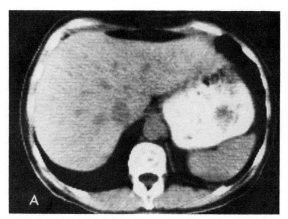

FIGURE 2–1a

The liver occupies most of the section. It does not have a homogeneous appearance. There are multiple small, round areas of decreased attenuation, especially centrally near the porta hepatis. There is also a larger area of decreased attenuation in the posterior medial aspect of the liver. The caudate lobe lies between this structure and the aorta. The stomach, filled with dilute contrast medium and food, and the spleen are also seen.

Now evaluate the second section.

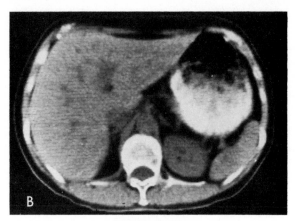

FIGURE 2–1b

The rounded areas of decreased attenuation in the liver branch and radiate from the liver hilus. There is a small area of even lower attenuation in the porta hepatis, which is fat.

What does the third section tell you?

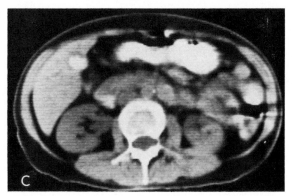

FIGURE 2–1c

The gallbladder has been opacified for the oral cholecystogram and has a higher attenuation than the surrounding liver parenchyma. Ordinarily the gallbladder is a low density structure because it contains bile, which has a high fat content.

What do you think the rounded and branching areas of decreased attenuation are? A dilated biliary system could have this appearance, since bile contains fat and has a lower attenuation than the surrounding liver. The bile ducts do radiate from the porta hepatis. Normal-sized bile ducts, however, are too small to be visualized and Mrs. B. R. is not jaundiced and has no clinical evidence of hepatobiliary disease.

The scans were repeated after an intravenous infusion of contrast material. The repeat scans solve the mystery. One scan is demonstrated.

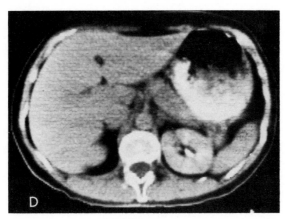

FIGURE 2-1d

In all the postinfusion scans, the low density areas seen before are virtually indistinguishable from the surrounding liver. This observation means that these structures are not dilated bile ducts, since bile would remain at its baseline density after intravenous infusion of contrast medium. These branching structures are the normal portal venous system and should not be confused with the biliary sytem, although their distribution is parallel. The large round low density area in the posterior medial aspect of the liver seen on the first scan is the hepatic segment of the inferior vena cava and also should not be confused with an abnormality. Portal vein visualization is not consistent but can be enhanced by a large intravenous infusion of contrast material.

Mrs. B. R. has no lymphoma demonstrated beyond the original site and responds well to therapy.

CASE 2–2:

NORMAL ANATOMY AND VARIATIONS

The configuration of the normal liver is highly variable. Some patients have almost no left lobe, others have a prominent Riedel's lobe extending well below the costal margin. The position of the liver also varies from patient to patient. As a rule, it will be lower in a patient with severe emphysema than in a patient with normal lungs. It is elevated with diaphragmatic elevation or eventration. All hepatic scans must be performed and interpreted with this in mind. Each examination must be designed for the individual problem and tailored by the scanning information as it is obtained. The first section illustrated was obtained at 2 cm below the tip of the xyphoid, a position usually well within liver. What do you see?

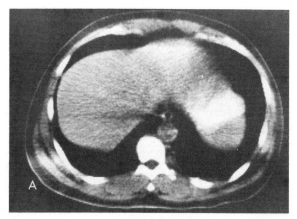

FIGURE 2–2a

The liver appears to be surrounded by air. In fact, this patient has severe chronic obstructive lung disease and the diaphragm is markedly depressed. What is actually seen here is some liver, some diaphragm, some stomach filled with contrast medium and possibly a bit of the spleen. An enlarged mediastinal node is also seen to the left of the spine and there is air in the esophagus. The artifacts are caused by cardiac motion. Useful information about the liver is rarely obtained on scans this high in the organ, though in a given case the attempt may be worthwhile.

The next scan, from another patient, was also obtained 2 cm below the xyphoid tip. What do you see?

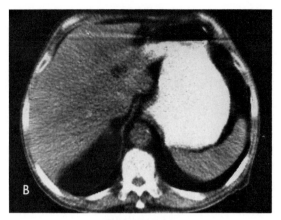

FIGURE 2-2b

This man's scan shows a good example of a generous right lobe of the liver with a small left one. The caudate lobe is somewhat prominent. Fat is seen in the porta hepatis. The stomach is rather large and its proximity to the aorta is an interesting observation. No significant abnormalities are present. Compare this scan with the next one done at a slightly lower level on another patient.

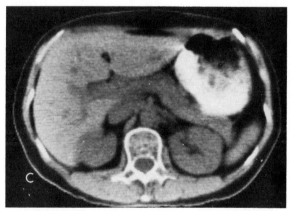

FIGURE 2-2c

This is another normal liver configuration but this woman has a larger left lobe and a smaller right one. The porta hepatis is prominent. In addition, the relationship of the liver to the kidneys and the pancreas is totally different from that in the first two cases. The crus of the right hemidiaphragm is forming the oval soft tissue density behind the inferior vena cava.

The next scan was made about 2 cm below the xyphoid. What do you see?

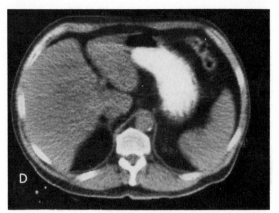

FIGURE 2–2d

The falciform ligament is seen in its entirety extending from the ventral surface of the liver to the porta hepatis. The round density in the porta hepatis is probably the portal vein, but studies enhanced by contrast medium would help in making this determination. In this patient, descending colon is situated between the stomach and abdominal wall. No colon is seen on scans *b* and *c*. A portion of the right adrenal gland is seen in the fat dorsal to the caudate lobe and inferior vena cava.

The final scan in this group was done about 6 cm below the xyphoid tip. What do you see?

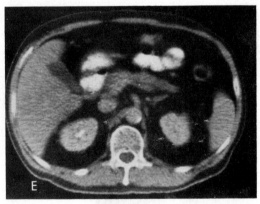

FIGURE 2–2e

At this level, the liver generally is positioned along the right lateral abdominal wall and can have innumerable configurations. The low density structure on the medial aspect of the liver is the gallbladder. Contrast medium in the duodenum outlines the head of the pancreas; the left adrenal gland is seen ventral to the left kidney.

Though this assortment of normal sections is small, it should give you an idea of the variability of the liver in configuration and location and in its relationships to other organs. All CT scans of the liver must be performed and interpreted with this in mind. A "routine" for examination of the liver based on external landmarks is not practical and so, for the cases that follow, such locations are generally not provided.

MRS. J. M.

Mrs. J. M. is referred for evaluation of episodic upper abdominal pain. Six years prior to her present illness she underwent cholecystectomy and common bile duct exploration for cholelithiasis with common duct obstruction. Initially she did well, but for the past six months she has complained of abdominal pain, nausea and vomiting. An upper gastrointestinal series and barium enema have been unrevealing; ultrasound was technically unsatisfactory and so a CT scan was ordered to evaluate the pancreas. The initial section was performed 3 cm below the xyphoid through the fundus and body of the stomach, which has been filled with dilute contrast material. What abnormality is present?

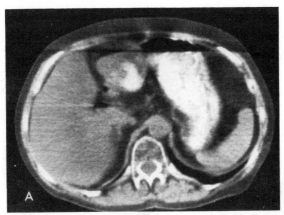

FIGURE 2–3a

Two small gas-filled structures of very low x-ray attenuation are seen in the porta hepatis. One is just below the cleft that contains the falciform ligament separating the lateral segment of the left lobe of the liver from the remainder of the liver. The other lies between the right lobe and the caudate lobe. These are gas-filled bile ducts that had been seen on routine x-rays. Incompetence of the ampulla of Vater has followed the common duct exploration. The spleen is seen against the diaphragm on the left. The close approximation of stomach and spleen is well seen. Branches of the celiac artery are ventral to the aorta.

The next section is 3 cm more caudal. What structures do you see?

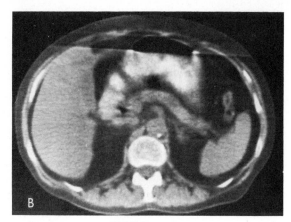

FIGURE 2–3b

The body and antrum of the stomach as well as the first portion of the duodenum are filled with contrast material. The body and tail of the pancreas are seen arching over the aorta and a portion of the head is also seen. The origin of the superior mesenteric artery is dorsal to the body of the pancreas and the left adrenal gland is dorsal to the pancreatic tail. The gas-filled common bile duct is seen between the duodenum and the head of the pancreas. The inferior vena cava is dorsal to the pancreatic head.

Mrs. J. M. has a horizontally oriented pancreas; this anatomical variation allows most of the organ to be studied in a single section. The presence of gas in the bile ducts allows visualization of the common bile duct, which cannot normally be separated from the pancreas and the duodenum.

The next section is 2 cm below the last. What structures are seen?

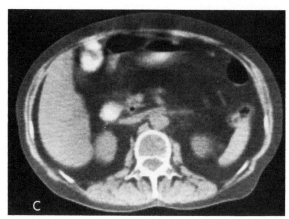

FIGURE 2–3c

A small portion of the pancreatic head is seen anterior to the inferior vena cava, which is collapsed. The left renal vein is seen crossing anterior to the aorta. Again, the gas-filled common bile duct is visualized posterior and to the right of the head of the pancreas. The second portion of the duodenum is filled with contrast medium. Posterior to this is the upper pole of the right kidney.

Mrs. J. M.'s pain continued to defy explanation. However, she is pleased to find that she does not have cancer and her symptoms gradually resolve.

MRS. D. R.

Over the years Mrs. D. R. has had several episodes of pancreatitis apparently caused by small gallstones in the common bile duct. Cholecystectomy and common duct exploration four years ago led to a cessation of these attacks. Many tiny stones were removed from the common bile duct at surgery however and you have just been waiting for trouble to recur. Mrs. D. R. comes in with abdominal pain that she feels is similar to her previous pancreatitis though not quite as bad. She has some abdominal tenderness and you wonder if she is jaundiced. You draw blood for a series of tests and send her for an ultrasound to look for dilated bile ducts and pancreatic abnormalities. No dilated intrahepatic ducts are seen and the pancreas cannot be examined satisfactorily because of bowel gas. Bilirubin is reported just barely elevated and serum amylase is about 300, a real but not major elevation.

Mrs. D. R. is anxious for a resolution of her problems, so you request an intravenous cholangiogram and within three hours receive a report from the radiologist. The common bile duct measures 15 mm, which he believes is upper limit of normal in a postcholecystectomy patient, and no stones are seen. Contrast material is seen entering the duodenum.

You discuss the diagnostic dilemma with the radiologist, who says that a CT scan may demonstrate the pancreas well even in the presence of bowel gas. After talking this over with Mrs. D. R. you schedule her for a CT scan late in the afternoon.

Aside from the contrast medium given about five hours earlier for the intravenous cholangiogram, no intravenous or oral contrast medium was given. The pancreas is normal and not fully demonstrated on these sections, which are selected to demonstrate the biliary system. What do you see on the first two scans?

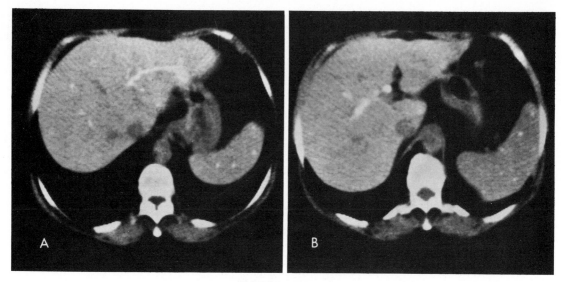

FIGURE 2–4a, b

These sections are so high in the abdomen that lung is included posteriorly. The spleen contains some punctate high attenuation densities, probably granulomata from previous infections. On scan *a* the left hepatic bile duct is seen filled with contrast material, while some of the right is seen on scan *b*. The central round duct is the common hepatic bile duct. The distribution of bile ducts parallels that of the portal veins. Opacification of one system or the other will aid in differentiation of the two during CT scanning when the question arises. The inferior vena cava is seen as a round, low attenuation structure within the liver near the aorta.

The next three scans demonstrate the course of the common bile duct from the porta hepatis into the head of the pancreas. Contrast medium is also present in the duodenum and small bowel from the intravenous cholangiogram.

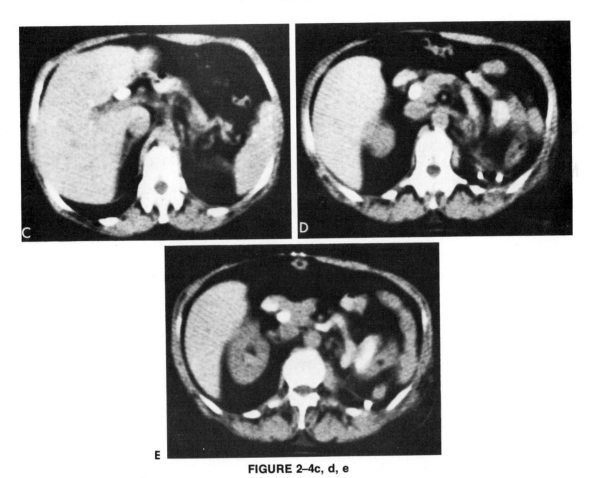

FIGURE 2–4c, d, e

The common bile duct is easy to see on these sections as it progresses medially and dorsally from the porta hepatis through the head of the pancreas toward the ampulla of Vater. It is larger than usual but probably within normal limits for a postcholecystectomy patient. On these scans you should make some interesting observations. The spleen is seen on *c*, which makes you wonder about enlargement, especially since the splenic tip may actually be seen on *d* lateral to a bowel loop. The superior mesenteric artery is seen arising from the aorta on *c*, and in cross section on *d*. Branches of the celiac artery to the liver and the spleen are seen on *c*. The left renal vein is seen crossing anterior to the aorta and entering the inferior vena cava on *d*. Both the right and the left adrenal glands are seen on *c*. The right one lies in the angle dorsal to the caudate lobe and the left is dorsal to the splenic artery.

Mrs. D. R.'s case is still an enigma, though her scans have been quite interesting to study. Her husband calls, concerned about the length of time she has been gone, and you learn that Mrs. D. R. has been drinking heavily for about nine months since her oldest son was killed in an automobile accident. Mrs. D. R. readily admits this. You arrange for her to visit the alcohol abuse clinic at your hospital after explaining the probable relationship between heavy drinking and her current physical problems. She seems relieved that someone has taken a positive step for her and follows through with her appointment. You see her a week later and things are going better.

CASE 2–5:

MS. K. H.

Ms. K. H. is a 29 year old woman with recently diagnosed Hodgkin's disease in an axillary node. You are in the process of staging her disease and order a CT scan to look for hepatosplenomegaly and retroperitoneal adenopathy. No evidence of Hodgkin's disease below the diaphragm is found but there is a striking abnormality.

The scans illustrated are all done without oral or intravenous contrast medium. What is unusual on all three scans?

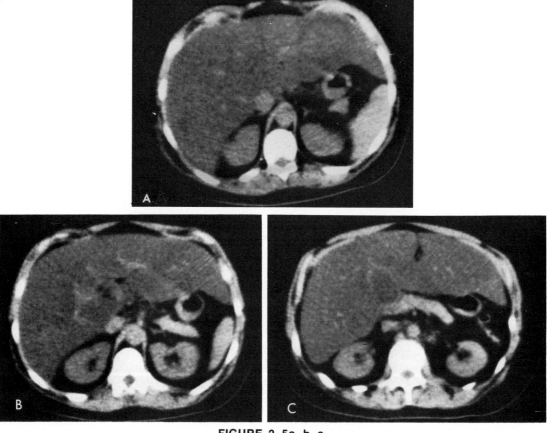

FIGURE 2–5a, b, c

The striking finding is the decreased attenuation of the liver substance when compared to the kidneys, spleen, pancreas, aorta and inferior vena cava. Normally, the liver has a higher attenuation than all of these structures, but here the relationship is reversed. In fact, the portal veins are seen within the liver substance without contrast medium infusion. Did you pick out the gallbladder on section *c*? It has almost the same attenuation as the liver substance.

By now you should have realized that Ms. K. H. has a fatty liver. Fatty liver is often an incidental finding because it is generally asymptomatic. Since it can be associated with alcohol abuse, you ask Ms. K. H. about her drinking habits. It seems she has always been a heavy social drinker, but concern about her Hodgkin's disease has led to several recent extended drinking sprees. You and her oncologist reassure her about her prognosis, pointing out that liver failure from drinking is a more serious threat to her life than the Hodgkin's disease, which is limited to the axilla.

CASE 2–6:

MRS. M. T.

Mrs. M. T. is no stranger to you. About five months ago you did a cholecystojejunostomy for decompression of obstructive jaundice caused by a carcinoma in the head of the pancreas. At that time the tumor was small but was firmly adherent to the superior mesenteric and portal veins so resection for cure was not feasible. Mrs. M. T.'s convalescence was complicated by an emotional collapse and she has been on a succession of medications for her depression. She comes in complaining of fatigue and malaise. You start to reassure her; then you notice she is somewhat jaundiced. You order a CT scan to differentiate a drug-induced cholestatic jaundice from extrahepatic obstructive jaundice. A single section through the liver is illustrated. What do you see?

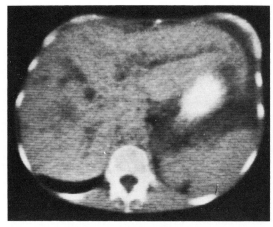

FIGURE 2–6

Massively dilated bile ducts are seen in both the right and left lobes of the liver. The portal veins have the same anatomic distribution but are rarely this large. Intravenous infusion of contrast medium will differentiate between the two systems when this question arises. On this section the aorta and the porta hepatis are obscured by added soft tissue which is undoubtedly tumor. The poorly defined low density area in the right lobe is a focus of metastatic carcinoma.

Little can be done for Mrs. M. T. since further decompression is not possible and her tumor is progressing rapidly. In fact, she undergoes a very rapid decline and dies a few weeks later. Postmortem examination demonstrates sheets of tumor extending into the porta hepatis and compressing the common hepatic bile duct.

When available, ultrasound can demonstrate dilated intrahepatic bile ducts very well and can often define the nature and level of the obstruction. It should be tried before CT in most patients.

MRS. S. M.

Mrs. S. M. is a 58 year old woman from the Philippines who comes to see you because her friends have told her that her eyes are yellow. She hasn't really felt well for some time but attributes that to nerves. On physical examination, you discover a right paramedian scar. She says she got that the last time she turned yellow about ten years ago at home. You order an ultrasound study because you suspect recurrent common duct stones. Dilated intrahepatic ducts are demonstrated and the proximal common bile duct is also dilated. Unfortunately, the distal common bile duct and head of the pancreas are obscured by bowel gas so you order a CT scan to look for a mass in the head of the pancreas or stones in the distal common bile duct.

The CT scan is done both before and after intravenous contrast medium is infused. The first two scans illustrated are done at about the same level before and after the infusion. What do you see?

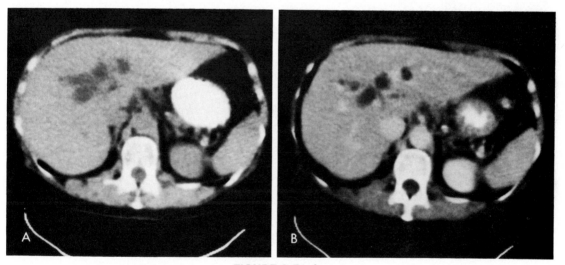

FIGURE 2–7a, b

The first thing that should strike you is the group of low attenuation structures located centrally in the liver. On scan b after contrast medium has been given, you can see the relationship of these structures to the portal veins and you should feel confident in identifying them as dilated intrahepatic bile ducts. The spleen and the tip of the left kidney are also seen on these cuts; also, the origin of the celiac artery from the aorta is demonstrated. The intrahepatic portion of the inferior vena cava can be seen on scan b.

The next three scans are done approximately 8, 10 and 12 cm distal to the first two. They are all done after the contrast medium infusion. What do you see?

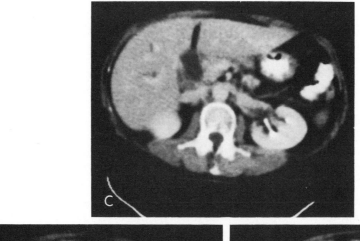

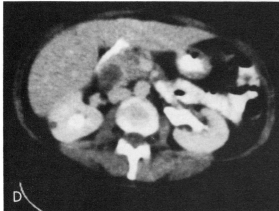
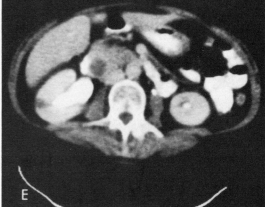

FIGURE 2–7c, d, e

Scan *c* shows a low density structure in the porta hepatis. Its orientation makes you think that it is the dilated common bile duct. The lower two sections show the dilated common bile duct in a normal sized pancreatic head. You do not see a calcified gallstone, but the absence of a pancreatic soft tissue mass increases the probability that Mrs. S. M. has recurrent stones. The fact that her gallbladder is never seen strengthens your belief that she had a cholecystectomy years ago.

There are some incidental findings on these last three scans. Did you identify the superior mesenteric artery and vein? They are best seen on scan *d* and are the two small round structures ventral to the aorta slightly to the left of midline. The vein is the larger structure. You should also have noticed the tiny cysts in the right kidney.

When you finally convince Mrs. S. M. that she should be operated upon, you find two large noncalcified stones in her distal common bile duct as well as fine gravel throughout the biliary system. You clean things up as much as possible, do a sphincterotomy and place a large T-tube in the common bile duct. However, you have few illusions of a cure.

MRS. L. C.

Mrs. L. C., a 55 year old nurse at your hospital, presents with epigastric pain. She gives a history of having eaten a fatty meal prior to the onset of her pain and also says she has had previous similar episodes. Gallbladder disease is suspected and an oral cholecystogram is ordered. This study is normal. Since the pain is somewhat colicky in nature, an intravenous urogram is ordered. The scout radiograph and the five minute film are shown. Does anything strike you as unusual, and if so, what is its significance?

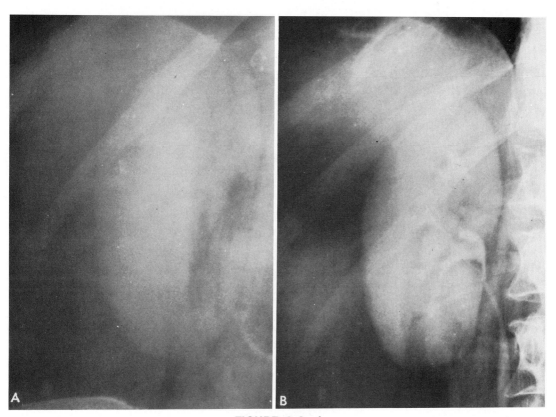

FIGURE 2–8a, b

The contour and collecting structures of the right kidney are normal. There is a rounded lucency in the liver. This is well seen on the film *b* done five minutes after the contrast medium injection, but it is also seen faintly on the scout film. This unusual lucency is now the focus of your attention. Most liver lesions are not seen as lucencies on x-ray; for this reason, a fatty mass is suggested. A CT scan is requested to evaluate the composition of the mass. What conclusions can be made from the CT scan?

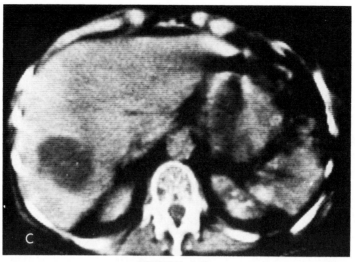

FIGURE 2–8c

There is a well defined homogeneous area of decreased attenuation in the right lobe of the liver corresponding to the lucency on the urogram. The CT number of the low density mass is +10, while that of the retroperitoneal fat is −162. All these facts suggest a simple cyst of the liver. What study would you do to confirm this impression?

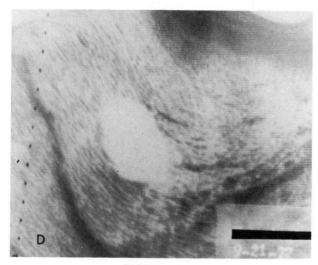

FIGURE 2–8d

The longitudinal ultrasound scan of the liver shows a well circumscribed transonic area with enhanced sound transmission. These findings, which indicate the presence of fluid, confirm the cystic nature of the hepatic lesion. The ability of ultrasound to differentiate fluid from solid lesions with great accuracy is a major advantage of this technique and makes it the procedure of choice for evaluation of suspected cysts.

It is thought unlikely that Mrs. L. C.'s symptoms are due to the simple liver cyst, and the following day a duodenal ulcer is found on the upper gastrointestinal series.

Computerized tomography is very sensitive to differences in tissue x-ray attenuation. Conventional radiographs are much less sensitive but will occasionally detect small differences as in this patient.

Mrs. R. S. is a vivacious 41 year old woman who had a left mastectomy three years ago. She has had regular followup visits and has had no
obvious recurrence of her tumor. At this visit she mentions some slight
weight loss and fatigue, so you order laboratory tests and a radionuclide
liver scan. All the blood tests are normal, but the isotopic examination is
not. What do you see on the posterior view from the scan?

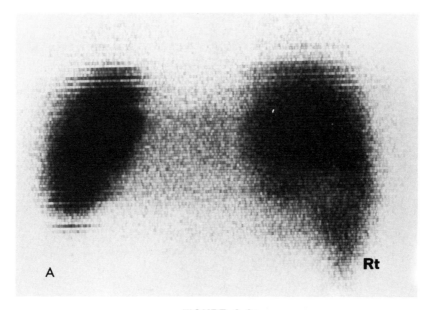

FIGURE 2–9a

An area of decreased uptake is present in the inferior medial aspect
of the right lobe of the liver. It is best seen on posterior view, indicating
that it is in the dorsal half of the liver. The finding seems to be new since
her preoperative scan three years ago, but because that examination was
performed on older equipment the studies are not comparable. The isoto-
pist is not dogmatic in his interpretation of the change but raises the
question of a solitary metastasis. An ultrasound is requested to get more
information about the lesion. With the patient supine, good definition of
the lesion is not obtained. Unfortunately, when the patient is turned
prone, the lesion lies immediately beneath a rib. The ultrasonographer
thinks the lesion is cystic but since you are planning to operate on the
lesion if it is a solitary metastasis, you decide to get a CT scan. What is
your conclusion?

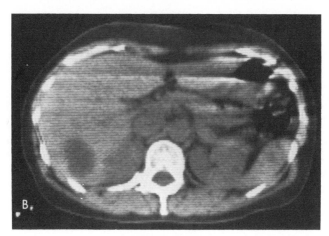

FIGURE 2–9b

There is a low attenuation mass in the dorsal portion of the right lobe of the liver that is sharply defined and rounded. The CT number of the mass is −7. The radiologist assures you that this is a simple hepatic cyst.

You are convinced that the mass is a cyst, but Mrs. R. S. has become alarmed by all the fancy tests she has undergone and will not rest until she knows for sure that the mass is not cancerous. The radiologist aspirates it for you under CT guidance. The sight of clear fluid and a negative cytology set Mrs. R. S.'s mind at rest.

MRS. P. C.

Mrs. P. C. is a 58 year old woman who has polycystic liver and kidney disease. Several family members have had a more severe form of the disease so Mrs. P. C. worries continually, and with some reason, about progression of her renal involvement. On this visit, however, she throws you a curve ball. She announces that she also has cysts in her pancreas and that they are now causing abdominal pain. What is more, she knows how you are going to prove her right! You are going to do one of those new scans that slices the whole body. You tell her that little useful knowledge about her condition will be gained from a CT scan. She marches out of your office in anger only to return about three weeks later with CT scans in hand. You were right—no practical information was obtained and the pancreas, though hard to see, seems to be normal. However, it is an interesting study, and so several scans are demonstrated. What do you see?

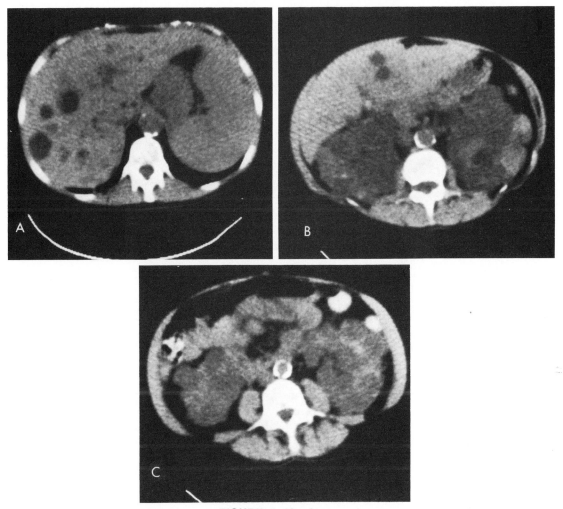

FIGURE 2–10a, b, c

On scan *a* the spleen is large but has no cysts. Many cysts of various sizes are seen in the liver. Some are rather poorly defined. Scans *b* and *c* show the markedly enlarged kidneys with many large and small cysts. The renal contours are classical for this disease, with many bulbous deformities caused by the cysts.

Mrs. P. C. is happy with her scans but does not tell you for many months how she managed to get them done. Later you learn that her daughter is an x-ray technologist in another state.

There is little indication for CT scanning in the patient with known polycystic renal disease. CT scanning is indicated following the discovery of large poorly functioning kidneys when plain films and ultrasound do not provide a definitive diagnosis. There may be a role for CT in the screening of family members. The examination by CT of an individual with known stable disease is unlikely to be productive.

Mr. Z. W. has a ten year history of gallstones and recurrent right upper quadrant pain but he has steadfastly refused surgery. Two weeks ago he began to have a fever and pain that was much more severe than usual. Finally his wife has forced him to see his doctor. A tender right upper quadrant mass is palpated and a radionuclide liver scan is obtained. What do you see?

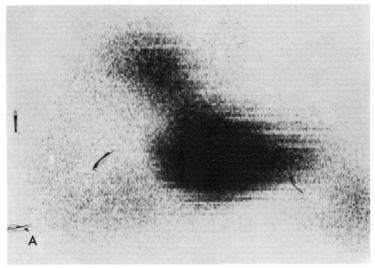

FIGURE 2–11a

A very large filling defect is present in the right lobe of the liver. A CT scan is ordered to try to characterize the abnormality more completely. The first section is at the level of the xyphoid. Is there any abnormality? Intravenous contrast medium has been given.

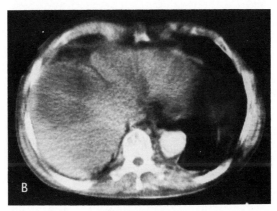

FIGURE 2–11b

There is significant motion artifact, since the patient is by now very ill and cannot suspend respiration. Even so, a large, round area of diminished attenuation can be seen in the anterior aspect of the right lobe of the liver. A septum appears to traverse the mass. Between the large lesion and the anterior abdominal wall a nonhomogeneous object of even lower attenuation is present.

The next section is 2 cm below the xyphoid. What do you find at this level?

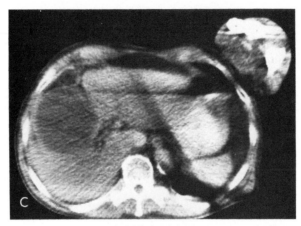

FIGURE 2–11c

The large area of decreased attenuation is again seen. Though the mass lies within the confines of the liver, it has a thick irregular wall and could be a lesion of extrahepatic origin that has burrowed into the liver. The area of lower attenuation is again seen ventral to the liver.

At the next level, 2 cm more caudal, what is seen?

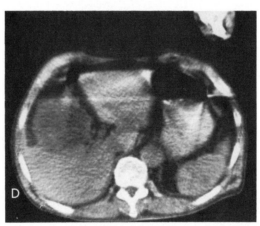

FIGURE 2–11d

At this level, the mass is more clearly extrahepatic and is displacing the right lobe of the liver dorsally. The thick irregular wall of the mass is better seen.

The gallbladder is not seen on these or any other sections. In view of the patient's long history of gallbladder disease and the current symptoms, hepatic abscess secondary to gallbladder rupture is the most likely diagnosis.

At surgery, a large abscess is found in the gallbladder fossa extending into the liver. The abscess is bordered by the diaphragm and the liver, which is adherent to the diaphragm. Anteriorly, the omentum is adherent to the inflammatory mass, causing the low attenuation area between the liver and the anterior abdominal wall. The inferior aspect of the abscess is formed by the remnant of the gallbladder, which had ruptured into the adjacent liver. A cholecystectomy is performed with extensive drainage of the abscess. The patient has an uneventful postoperative course.

Ms. M. H. is an adventurous 28 year old woman who has been your patient since childhood. This time she appears in your office looking quite ill and complaining of intermittent fever and upper abdominal distress. She has lost some weight but attributes that to severe bouts of diarrhea and poor appetite she had while backpacking in Mexico. You examine her and wonder if her bilirubin is elevated. Her liver is definitely enlarged and quite tender. All in all, you think Ms. M. H. has gotten hepatitis, but you order a radionuclide scan along with the blood chemistries to make sure you are missing nothing. The radionuclide scan report horrifies you. What is seen on this anterior view?

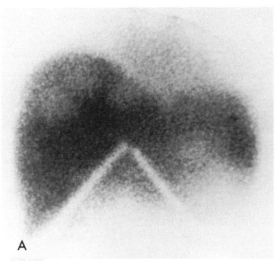

FIGURE 2–12a

There are several peripheral areas of diminished uptake of the radionuclide in both lobes of the liver. The report suggests multiple metastases. You know that there must be another explanation for the filling defects and question Ms. M. H. more closely about her travels and illnesses. It seems she has spent many months in Mexico and Central America and has had several tiresome bouts of cramping diarrhea with bloody mucus. Since returning home she has been tired and has had vague aches and pains. Suddenly you recall your former parasitology professor and suspect amebiasis. Stool examination confirms your idea and you decide to get a CT scan of the liver to better identify all the hepatic lesions. One scan done prior to infusion of intravenous contrast medium and two done after are illustrated. What do you see?

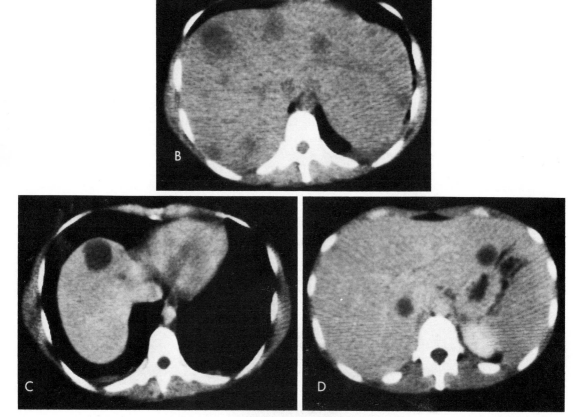

FIGURE 2–12b, c, d

Scan *b*, done prior to contrast medium infusion, demonstrates at least six rather poorly defined rounded, low attenuation areas in the liver. Following contrast medium infusion, cuts at two other levels give a somewhat better picture of similar lesions but there is no enhancement of either the lesions or their margins by the contrast medium. Scan *c* shows two interesting findings. First, there are small bilateral pleural effusions, a common finding in hepatic amebic abscess. Second, one abscess is located immediately beneath the liver capsule adjacent to the diaphragm. One complication of hepatic amebic abscess is spread of the abscess to the thorax caused by rupture of the liver lesion through the diaphragm. It is easy to imagine such an occurrence in this patient.

Ms. M. H. responds well to antiamebic therapy. Resolution of her abscesses is observed primarily by radionuclide scans. However, to be sure the abscesses have completely resolved, a CT scan is ordered before she leaves on a jaunt to Afghanistan.

The nonspecific nature of CT scanning in the liver is emphasized here. In this patient more lesions could be seen by CT scanning than by radionuclide scan, but the nature of the lesions was not determined by CT. Since more lesions were demonstrated on the initial CT scan than by isotopic scan, it was useful as the final arbiter of successful therapy.

Mrs. G. W., a 71 year old woman who has recently immigrated from Hong Kong, seeks medical attention because of a mass in the right upper abdomen. She speaks only broken English but says she has had "liver trouble" for many years. The mass and some right upper quadrant pain began only two months ago and have steadily increased. An enlarged firm liver is palpated and a ⁹⁹ᵐTc sulfur colloid liver scan is obtained. What do you see?

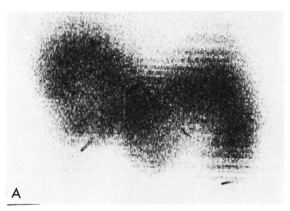

FIGURE 2-13a

A large filling defect that suggests a hepatoma is present in the right lobe of the liver. Both the liver and spleen are enlarged. The patient's serum liver chemistries are abnormal and an alpha-1-fetoglobulin is markedly elevated. A CT scan is ordered to assess the extent of the suspected hepatoma before a decision is made about appropriate surgical or medical therapy.

The initial section at 1 cm below the xyphoid tip is done prior to intravenous contrast medium infusion. Do you see any abnormality?

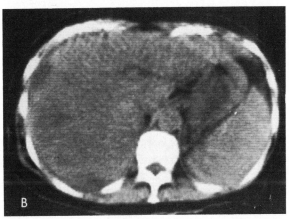

FIGURE 2-13b

The liver is large and the left lobe extends almost to the left lateral abdominal wall. The spleen is also enlarged. The fundus of the stomach is seen between the left lobe of the liver and the spleen. The liver has a rather homogeneous internal consistency except for the posterolateral aspect of the right lobe, which is mottled. This section is repeated after contrast medium infusion. Can you see any change?

45

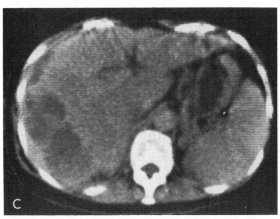

FIGURE 2–13c

It is readily apparent that the area of abnormal attenuation in the liver is much more extensive and better demonstrated than on the scan done without contrast medium. Much of the tumor has attenuation characteristics similar to the surrounding liver and cannot be identified without contrast medium enhancement of the normal liver. Such an improvement in visualization emphasizes the role of contrast medium in the CT examination of the liver. Since it is also possible to bring a lesion up to the same density as the surrounding liver tissue, scans of the liver must be obtained prior to and after contrast medium infusion in most cases.

The next section was obtained 5 cm below the first two at the level of the kidneys. What further information do you obtain?

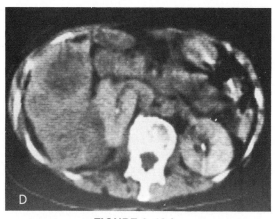

FIGURE 2–13d

In this section the mottled areas of decreased attenuation in the liver can be seen to involve the entire inferior aspect of the right lobe. On the posterior medial aspect of the liver, tumor can be seen bulging from the liver into the retroperitoneal fat. The fat plane between the liver and the kidney is obliterated, and the right kidney is deformed and displaced ventrally and medially. The inferior vena cava is displaced by the right kidney.

Percutaneous needle biopsy confirms the diagnosis of hepatoma. The extent of the mass beyond the confines of the liver makes the hepatoma unresectable for cure. An angiogram is obtained during placement of a catheter in the common hepatic artery for direct arterial perfusion chemotherapy.

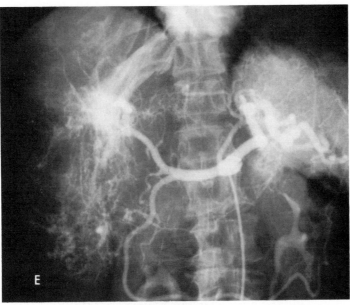

FIGURE 2–13e

The celiac angiogram shows extensive tumor neovascularity in the right lobe. The right hepatic vein is invaded by tumor and is well opacified by shunted contrast material, confirming the CT diagnosis of nonresectability.

Mrs. G. W. does not survive long, dying of hepatic failure. Since the only real chance for long-term survival in hepatoma is resection, use of CT scanning spared her a fruitless exploratory laparotomy.

CASE 2–14:

MRS. S. L.

Mrs. S. L. comes in for a semiannual followup examination. She feels well but complains of tiredness. Her mastectomy scar is unchanged and the slight arm swelling has disappeared since her previous visit. On physical examination, however, you palpate an enlarged liver. Her liver chemistries are abnormal and a ^{99m}Tc-sulfur colloid liver scan is obtained the next day. What do you see?

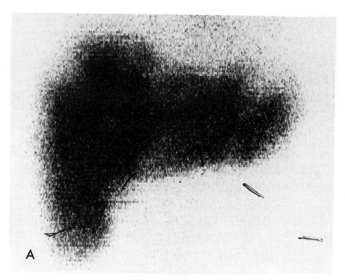

FIGURE 2–14a

Several round areas of non-uptake of the radioisotope are present. The most likely diagnosis is multiple liver metastases in view of her breast carcinoma, but other processes such as multiple cysts or abscesses could produce this pattern. Because of other vague abdominal symptoms, a CT scan is ordered. A single section through the upper abdomen is shown. What do you see? Intravenous contrast material has been given.

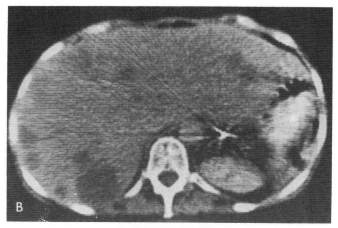

FIGURE 2–14b

There are many round areas of decreased attenuation in the liver. This organ virtually fills the upper abdomen. The high density point behind the left lobe is a metallic surgical clip. The CT number of the liver lesions is well above that of fluid, supporting the diagnosis of metastases. A needle biopsy confirms this diagnosis and intraarterial chemotherapy is begun when no other metastases are demonstrated.

It is apparent that little additional useful information is obtained by performing both radionuclide and CT scans in the evaluation of liver metastases when the radionuclide scan is positive. Though each method has advantages, the nuclide scan remains the basic screening test for metastases to the liver. When the radionuclide scan is inconclusive, CT may have a role in these patients.

The CT scan appearance seen in this case is representative of most cases of liver metastasis. These lesions are of lower attenuation than the surrounding liver and in general do not enhance as much as the liver when intravenous contrast medium infusion is given. Therefore, they are better seen on studies done after administration of contrast medium. Necrosis, hemorrhage or calcification all occur in metastatic foci and can alter this appearance.

CASE 2–15:

MRS. B. C.

Mrs. B. C. is a charming 57 year old woman who had a mucinous adenocarcinoma of the right colon resected about 15 months ago. You have been following her closely because several nodes in the resected specimen were positive for carcinoma. The report of a radionuclide liver scan suggests diffuse abnormality in the right hepatic lobe. Mrs. B. C. does not want to have a percutaneous liver biopsy and also does not wish to wait a few weeks for a followup radionuclide scan, so you decide together that a CT scan should be performed. Scanning is performed before and after an infusion of intravenous contrast material. What do you see on the first scan?

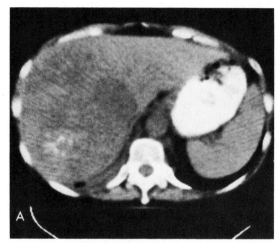

FIGURE 2–15a

The first section shows a mottled low attenuation region in the right lobe of the liver. Some well defined, punctate high density areas are also present. At this point, you should know the outcome of the study. The second scan was done after contrast medium had been given.

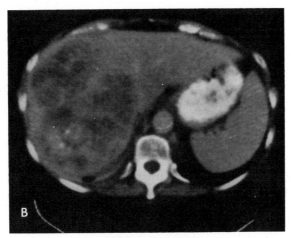

FIGURE 2–15b

The mottled low density region is seen to be several rounded lesions and the high density regions are unchanged.

Sadly, you can tell Mrs. B. C. that she does have multiple metastases in her liver. The high density regions are calcifications in the metastases, not an uncommon finding in mucinous adenocarcinoma. Such calcifications can often be seen on plain films, though Mrs. B. C.'s were not visible.

An incidental finding on these sections is the presence of enlarged retrocrural nodes immediately adjacent to the aorta. These are further evidence of metastases.

Mrs. B. C. is placed on chemotherapy and initially does well but expires eight months later.

CASE 2–16:

MRS. H. E.

Mrs. H. E. is a 70 year old woman who has been in good health most of her life and has generally avoided medical attention. She comes to see you after an interval of several years, saying she just doesn't feel well. She tires easily and has pain in her abdomen and a sensation of fullness. Her appetite is poor. Physical examination confirms her story. She has lost about 30 pounds without dieting and looks wasted. More distressing, her liver is markedly enlarged and you think you can feel her spleen. She also has enlarged, firm nodes in both groins. Mrs. H. E. is not a very cooperative patient and you fear she will not complete the lengthy series of laboratory and radiographic examinations that would constitute a logical approach to her problems so, after drawing blood for SMA panel, you arrange for an abdominal CT scan that afternoon. The study is done before and after an intravenous infusion of contrast material and covers the abdomen from xyphoid to symphysis pubis. Two sections through the liver are illustrated. What do you see on the first one?

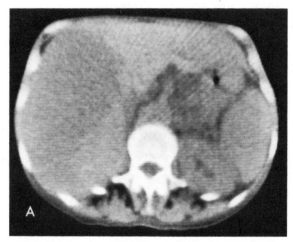

FIGURE 2–16a

The liver is enlarged on this section, a finding confirmed by the remainder of the examination. There is an extensive mottled low attenuation area involving primarily the right hepatic lobe. This is confluent but irregular in contour, suggesting an infiltrating lesion. The second scan was done after intravenous contrast medium infusion. What do you see now?

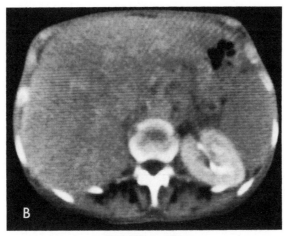

FIGURE 2–16b

Following contrast medium infusion, portal vein radicles are seen but the mass is less well defined. On both these sections a suggestion of abnormal nodes is seen lying between the aorta and superior mesenteric artery and the left kidney. Adenopathy is clearly present on lower sections. What is your diagnosis?

By now, you should realize that many lesions in the liver look rather similar. The possibilities in this patient, however, are relatively limited. She has no history to suggest an inflammatory process and focal cirrhosis is also very unlikely, since she does not drink and cirrhosis does not cause adenopathy. Neoplasm is therefore most likely. Metastases to the retroperitoneal nodes and the liver could look like this, though the solitary, central, infiltrating appearance of the liver mass is not typical of the more common metastases to liver.

Primary liver tumors for all practical purposes do not cause retroperitoneal adenopathy. Therefore, you should wonder about the lymphomas, placing this type of neoplasm at the top of your differential list, since not uncommonly it produces an infiltrating pattern of organ involvement. In fact, inguinal node biopsy and a percutaneous liver biopsy in this case both reveal Hodgkin's disease.

CHAPTER
3

CT SCANNING
OF THE PANCREAS

The pancreas is a difficult organ to evaluate with conventional radiographic techniques. Plain films will demonstrate calcifications in the pancreas and large masses may be detected. An upper gastrointestinal series is also of limited value, since more than half of all pancreatic masses are missed by this study. No successful radioisotopic examination has been devised. Angiography in experienced hands is highly informative, but it is an expensive, lengthy, invasive procedure with definite chance of patient morbidity. Endoscopic retrograde pancreatography, also invasive, is a technique that is not generally available. Ultrasound is the exception. It is an excellent modality for studying the pancreas and is limited only by the presence of bowel gas and marked obesity of the patient.

Computerized tomography demonstrates the entire pancreas, the surrounding peripancreatic fat and all adjacent organs. It is useful in evaluating local and diffuse changes of pancreatic size and attenuation. Masses that do not produce localized enlargement or a change in the x-ray attenuation will be difficult to detect. The peripancreatic fat is a great help in evaluating the gland itself, since it delineates the organ from surrounding structures. Infiltration of the fat is an important finding in pancreatic malignancies, though edema and blood can also obliterate the fat planes. In asthenic or emaciated patients with poorly developed fat planes, it is difficult to separate the pancreas from surrounding structures.

The major role of pancreatic CT scanning at present is in identification and evaluation of masses. These generally cause focal enlargements of the gland. Necrotic, calcified or hemorrhagic tumors have areas of altered attenuation, but otherwise, neoplasms have about the same attenuation as the normal pancreas. The obliteration of fat planes, vascular involvement, hepatic metastases and extension into mesentery or adjacent viscera are all signs of nonresectability for cure that may be seen on the CT scan. Dilated bile ducts may be seen in the liver when obstruction is caused by a mass in the head of the pancreas.

Inflammatory masses such as pseudocysts or abscesses have areas of decreased attenuation and sometimes gas. Without the clinical history it is often impossible to differentiate a pancreatic pseudocyst from an abscess or even a necrotic tumor. Calcifications, especially curvilinear ones, and a peripancreatic location make pseudocyst more likely. When pancreatic tumors obstruct the pancreatic ducts, pseudocysts and pancreatitis often result, so that several types of pathology are seen in the same patient. This means that it is important to pay close attention to subtle differences in attenuation and observe details such as wall thickness and regularity when evaluating CT scans of the pancreas.

Unless the patient is known to have large amounts of bowel gas or is very obese, ultrasound should be the primary technique in the evaluation of the pancreas. In about two-thirds of patients, ultrasound will be successful in obtaining good diagnostic information about the pancreas and CT scanning can be avoided. When a satisfactory ultrasound is not obtained, CT should be performed. When evaluation of peripancreatic spread of a neoplasm is of concern, CT should generally be the primary diagnostic technique.

CASE 3–1:

NORMAL PANCREAS AND VARIATIONS

CT is uniquely capable of evaluating the pancreas but care is needed both in performing and in interpreting the CT examination. The configuration of the pancreas is variable, though it usually takes a diagonal course across the abdomen with the tail positioned cephalad of the head. The pancreatic head is generally bulkier than the body and tail and there is often thinning of the body anterior to the spine.

Anatomic landmarks help in identifying the pancreas. The superior mesenteric artery arises from the aorta dorsal to the body of the pancreas. The uncinate process of pancreas may lie dorsal to the superior mesenteric artery slightly more distally but the bulk of the pancreas is ventral to this artery. The head of the pancreas lies in the duodenal sweep and bowel contents or oral contrast medium can define this separation well. The third or transverse portion of the duodenum may be confused with pancreas. Oral contrast medium aids in this differentiation. Identification of the superior mesenteric artery and vein ventral to the structure in question also is useful in determining that what is seen is duodenum.

The pancreas is generally surrounded by a layer of fat that helps to define its margins. However, the splenic vein is usually intimately related to the pancreatic tail, and the common bile duct and the portal vein may appear to add bulk to the pancreatic head. Emaciated patients may have insufficient fat for visualization, and pathological processes including edema, inflammation and neoplastic invasion may completely obscure the fat.

With these guidelines in mind, have a look at the scans that follow. The pancreas is normal in each case. You should try to identify the pancreas on each scan and observe its relationship to other organs.

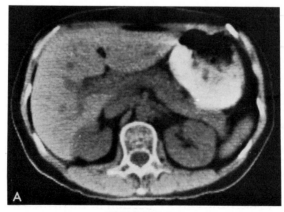

FIGURE 3–1a

This woman has a nearly transverse orientation of the pancreas. The tip of the tail is lying in the splenic hilum and the tail itself appears to be draped over the left kidney. It is easy to imagine how enlargement of either the spleen or the left kidney could displace the pancreas. The superior mesenteric artery has just arisen from the aorta, and body of the pancreas is ventral to it. The left renal vein is crossing anterior to the aorta to join the inferior vena cava. At this point, it becomes difficult to separate the pancreas from portal structures and the inferior vena cava. You should expect the head of the pancreas to be visualized on more caudal sections.

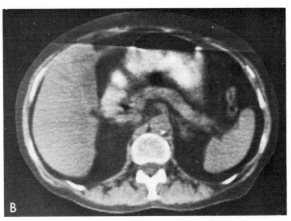

FIGURE 3–1b

This is a patient whose case you reviewed in Chapter 2. She has an incompetent sphincter at the ampulla of Vater and there is air in the common bile duct. This scan nicely identifies the head of the pancreas that is further delineated by contrast material in the duodenum. The body of the pancreas arcs over the origin of the superior mesenteric artery and the tail extends toward the spleen. Look carefully at the tail. Part of the splenic vein is seen distally adjacent to the pancreatic tail. In this particular patient the pancreas is cephalad to the left kidney but the left adrenal gland is seen dorsal to the pancreatic tail.

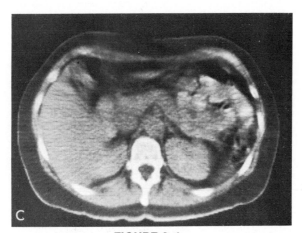

FIGURE 3–1c

In this patient only the central portion of the pancreas is seen at this level. The body merges with the inferior vena cava on the right, though the two have slightly differing attenuation numbers and can therefore be distinguished. On the left the tail merges with small bowel filled with contrast medium. Several additional sections were needed to complete the pancreatic examination.

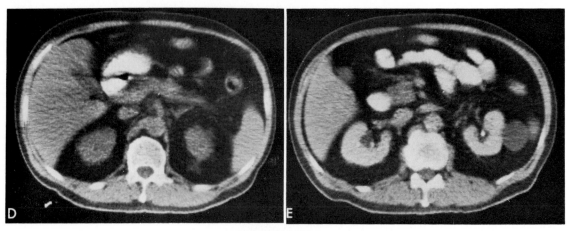

FIGURE 3–1d, e

These sections were done 3 cm apart. On *d* you may think that you are seeing the pancreatic head outlined by contrast medium in the descending duodenum. The inferior vena cava, superior mesenteric artery and left adrenal all can be seen; this helps to assure you that you are seeing the pancreas. The lower section, however, should catch your attention; on this scan the bulk of the pancreatic head is located medial to the descending duodenum. The superior mesenteric artery and vein are medial to it. The left renal vein is crossing anterior to the aorta to join the inferior vena cava. It is important to be sure you encompass the entire organ on your study and also to construct a three-dimensional image of the organ in your mind before drawing conclusions about shape and size.

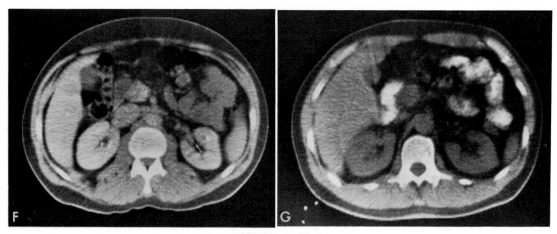

FIGURE 3–1f, g

In both of these patients, only the pancreatic head is seen on the section illustrated. In scan *f* the duodenum is fluid filled; in *g* it is filled with contrast material. In *f* the patient's Valsalva maneuver markedly expanded the inferior vena cava; in *g* it is quite small.

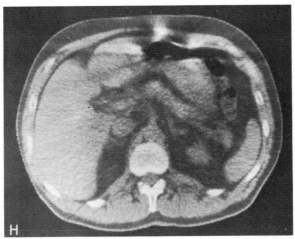

FIGURE 3–1h

This should be an easy case. You are seeing only the distal body and proximal tail of the pancreas with the splenic vein extending laterally from the tail. What did you call the soft tissue structures ventral to the inferior vena cava? These are the hepatic artery and portal vein along with the common bile duct. In this patient it is not possible to separate these structures, but none of it is pancreatic head; this is encountered more caudally.

The pancreas is obviously highly variable in position and configuration and it can be displaced by masses in adjacent organs. When a pancreatic CT scan is done, it is important to be sure that the entire gland has been studied.

CASE 3–2:

MR. J. F.

Mr. J. F. is a patient you will evaluate in detail later in this book (Case 4–9), since his primary problem is renal in nature. However, an observation about the pancreas can be made on this scan, which was done after both oral and intravenous contrast material had been given. What are your thoughts?

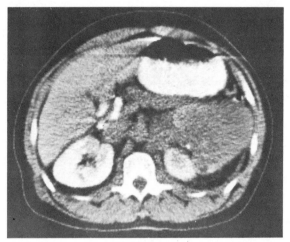

FIGURE 3–2

There is a large mass adjacent to the left kidney, which displaces the aorta to the right and pushes the tail of the pancreas ventrally, markedly thinning the normal fat planes and apparently compressing the pancreas. There is no intrinsic abnormality of the pancreas.

The pancreas is a retroperitoneal organ and is commonly thought to be rather immobile. This is incorrect, a fact that is often demonstrated at ultrasound and is now seen with CT scanning. Adjacent masses tend to stretch, thin and displace the pancreas, but splenomegaly, for example, may push the pancreatic tail medially, making it appear bulky, simulating a neoplasm. These secondary effects on the pancreas must be considered in the interpretation of pancreatic abnormalities in the presence of other pathology.

Loss of pliability of the pancreas may at times be a sign of pancreatic fibrosis or neoplastic infiltration. Pliability can be evaluated by doing a scan of the pancreas when the patient is in the right lateral decubitus position. Changes in pancreatic configuration with position indicate pliability.

Mrs. A. T. is a 50 year old woman who comes to your office for the first time looking very ill, in fact so ill that your secretary gets her into an examining room without delay. Her husband confides that she has a "drinking problem."

It seems that she has severe epigastric pain, especially in the left upper quadrant which radiates to her back. She has been vomiting uncontrollably for nearly a day. She has a low grade fever and says she has had some chills. On physical examination her abdomen is soft and there is no guarding. There is mild tenderness in the epigastrium and bowel sounds are diminished. You are sure she has acute pancreatitis; blood and urine amylase determinations confirm this diagnosis. You hospitalize her and start medical therapy, expecting improvement over a few days. However, after seeming to improve immediately after hospitalization, she again feels worse and her amylase rises. You wonder if she is developing a pancreatic pseudocyst and order an ultrasound. Bowel gas makes this examination technically unsatisfactory so you order a CT scan. Two sections are illustrated. Both are done after intravenous contrast medium has been given. What abnormalities do you see?

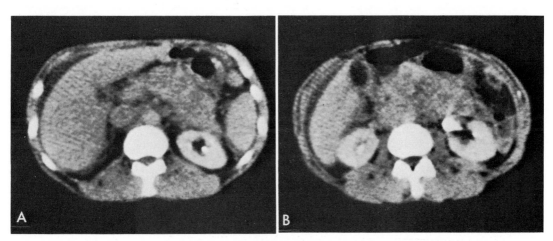

FIGURE 3–3a, b

Both scans show a very much enlarged pancreas, which has a mottled appearance often seen in acute pancreatitis. Scan *b* shows obliteration of the fat plane that is normally present between the aorta and the pancreas. This obliteration is generally caused by tumors but can also be caused by inflammation and edema. In the emaciated patient, the fat plane may be hard to see. No pancreatic pseudocysts are demonstrated but there is some ascites primarily located between the liver and the lateral abdominal wall. The gallbladder is seen on scan *b* as an ovoid low attenuation structure in the right lobe of the liver. Bowel gas is present in the transverse colon ventral to the pancreas. Such gas collections make ultrasound of the pancreas technically impossible.

On your evening visit to Mrs. A. T. you discover that she is drinking gin; she tells you she always drinks gin in the evening. You once again explain the connection between pancreatitis and alcohol and remove her bottle. She agrees to abstain for the moment "as a trial" and over the next days does begin to improve.

Mr. J. C. is an alcoholic with recurrent bouts of pancreatitis that generally follow prolonged heavy drinking. He has had several pseudocysts in the past so when his family brings him in to see you, their story does not surprise you. It seems that Mr. J. C. celebrated his 62nd birthday ten days ago by drinking more than a fifth of cheap gin and followed that by steady drinking for seven days until he developed nausea, vomiting and severe abdominal pain. As the nausea and vomiting increased, the drinking decreased. His family thinks Mr. J. C. has had no alcohol for 48 hours, and he does seem rather shaky.

Physical examination reveals a sallow, dehydrated, tremulous patient with abdominal fullness and moderate tenderness. When the emergency serum amylase you have ordered is reported at 2300 units, you admit Mr. J. C. with a diagnosis of pancreatitis and probable pseudocyst. Further diagnostic procedures seem unnecessary. Everything goes well with conservative therapy for pancreatitis and alcohol withdrawal until you notice that Mr. J. C. is becoming jaundiced and find that his bilirubin has risen to 5 mg% with an obstructive picture. You are faced with differentiating a cholestatic jaundice secondary to alcoholic hepatitis from extrahepatic obstructive jaundice. Since the patient has a persistent ileus, you decide to order a CT scan rather than an ultrasound. Three sections are illustrated. What do you see on the first one?

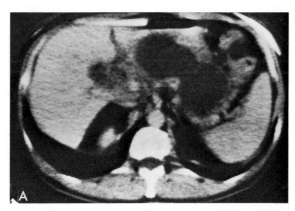

FIGURE 3–4a

The most dramatic abnormality is a dumbbell-shaped area of low attenuation in the tail of the pancreas, which you are sure is pancreatic pseudocyst. In addition, the spleen is moderately large and the porta hepatis is prominent with suggestion of dilated biliary ducts. The tip of the right kidney is seen. What information does the next scan add?

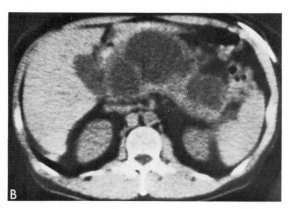

FIGURE 3–4b

The pancreatic pseudocyst has several locules and the pancreatic head is involved. The walls of the pseudocyst are somewhat irregular and the contents are not entirely homogeneous. The base of the gallbladder is seen and is large. No dilated intrahepatic bile ducts are seen at this level.

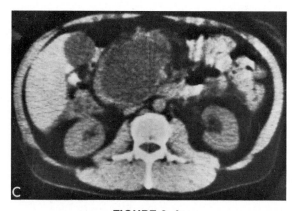

FIGURE 3–4c

The final scan shows a very large pseudocyst in the pancreatic head; the gallbladder is enlarged. The pseudocyst in the pancreatic head and the associated pancreatitis could certainly cause common bile duct obstruction. Since you see no dilated intrahepatic ducts, however, you cannot prove this hypothesis.

You decide that conservative care is best, since Mr. J. C. refuses a liver biopsy and he gradually improves. His pain diminishes and his serum amylase decreases. Followup ultrasound scans several weeks later show marked decrease in size of the pseudocyst in the pancreatic head and some decrease of the others. Mr. J. C.'s bilirubin returns to normal.

When your nurse tells you that Mrs. J. S. has arrived in your office without an appointment, you are sure of what you are about to hear. She has chronic relapsing pancreatitis and often shows up with severe abdominal pain. You are nearly correct; her complaint is pain, but now you also feel an epigastric mass. Her bowel sounds are diminished. You think she has an associated ileus, so you decide to skip an ultrasound examination of her pancreas and go straight to a CT scan. A single cut, which includes most of the pancreas, is shown. What do you see?

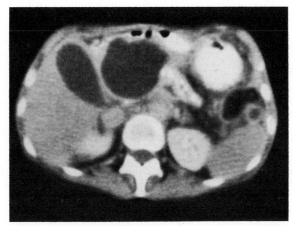

FIGURE 3–5

The stomach is filled with dilute Gastrografin and the antrum is draped over a large pseudocyst involving the head and body of the pancreas. This pseudocyst has rather smooth walls and homogeneous contents. Pseudocysts often have irregular walls and the contents can be mixed. Mrs. J. S. also has a string of calcifications in the pancreatic tail, which is thin and probably atrophic. A single calcification is seen in the wall of the pseudocyst. The fat planes between the pancreas and the aorta and the inferior vena cava are thinned but are still present. The dilatation of the gallbladder suggests obstruction of the common bile duct by the pseudocyst. The serum bilirubin is mildly elevated and other CT sections demonstrate some dilatation of intrahepatic ducts.

You decide to hospitalize Mrs. J. S. to tide her over the acute exacerbation of pancreatitis and to follow the progress of the pseudocyst. Most of her symptoms disappear with conservative therapy during the next few days and even the pseudocyst seems smaller. When the ileus resolves, you have followup studies done of the pseudocyst with ultrasound. Over the next few weeks it does diminish in size.

CASE 3–6:

MRS. A. L.

Mrs. A. L. is an elderly woman who has been having recurrent severe upper abdominal pain. Her concerned daughter says that the patient has been drinking heavily since the death of her husband two years ago. On physical examination she has a vague right upper quadrant mass, and her internist orders an upper gastrointestinal examination. The preliminary film and an oblique film of the filled stomach are shown. Do you see any abnormality?

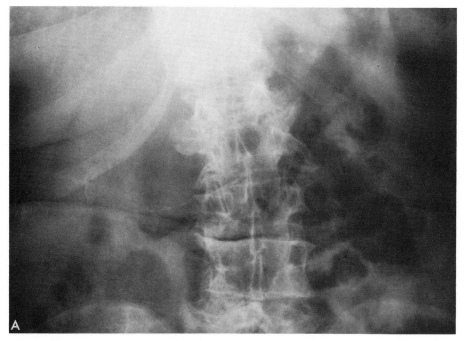

FIGURE 3–6a

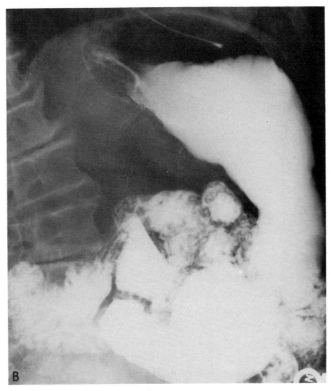

FIGURE 3–6b

On the preliminary film, there is an unusual curvilinear calcification to the right of the spine, as well as some scattered punctate calcifications in the same area. When the stomach is filled with barium, a mass effect is noted on the posterior aspect of the proximal portion of the duodenal sweep. These are all subtle observations. A CT scan is requested to further evaluate the mass in the right upper quadrant. A single section from the CT study is shown. Does this examination confirm the presence of a mass?

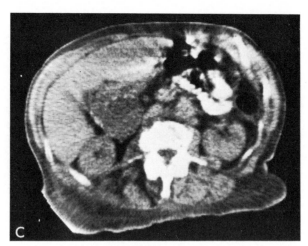

FIGURE 3–6c

There is an ovoid mass posterior to the liver and medial to the right kidney, which has several curvilinear calcifications in its wall. The internal structure of the mass is rather homogeneous and has a somewhat lower attenuation than that of the liver or kidney. Because the mass is located adjacent to the pancreas and because of its cystic appearance, the diagnosis of a pancreatic pseudocyst is made. An ultrasound examination is performed and the cystic mass is again demonstrated.

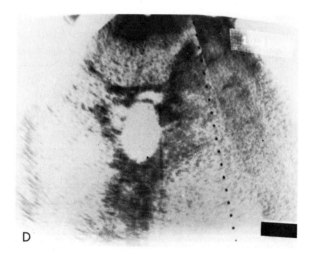

FIGURE 3–6d

After much debate, surgery is decided upon and a pancreatic pseudocyst is found. While other lesions such as cystadenoma might be considered in this patient, pancreatic pseudocyst is the most likely CT diagnosis.

CT certainly will demonstrate most pancreatic pathology very well, but ultrasound should generally be attempted first. It is simpler and more versatile. A certain number of patients will not be good ultrasound subjects, because of body habitus or bowel gas. It is sometimes possible to recognize these problems in advance and go straight to the CT scan. In the majority of patients, however, ultrasound will provide as much information as the CT scan and should be used first.

MR. R. S.

Mr. R. S. is a 28 year old hard-living construction worker who is a problem patient. Somehow he always has an atypical presentation of a common disorder and you are not happy to have him appear complaining of right flank pain. Though his urinalysis is normal, you order an intravenous urogram, which shows only displacement of the right kidney laterally. Ultrasound demonstrates a mass adjacent to the spine; the mass is nonhomogeneous but rather transonic. It does not demonstrate the head of the pancreas, though the body and tail are well seen and are normal.

Mr. R. S. is following his usual pattern and you question the patient and his family about events in the past few weeks. There is nothing out of the ordinary for Mr. R. S.: he has fallen out of scaffolding but only about ten feet; he was in a minor car wreck but walked away; and he had done some heavy drinking once or twice.

His back pain has increased over the past few days and he says he can't work so you hospitalize him and do a series of laboratory tests. Most of the results are normal but his serum amylase is 1800. When you repeat it, it comes back markedly elevated again. There is still no abdominal tenderness, but you believe Mr. R. S. must have a pseudocyst, possibly from trauma. A CT scan is performed. What do you see on the first section?

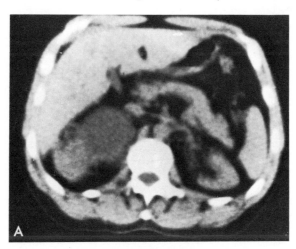

FIGURE 3–7a

The body and tail of the pancreas are well seen and are normal. A round, thick-walled, low attenuation mass is displacing the right kidney laterally. The mass is inseparable from the kidney on this section. What observations do you make on the second section?

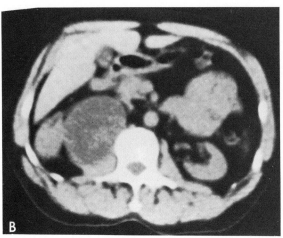

FIGURE 3–7b

The mass is larger at this level but continues to have a thick irregular wall. It seems to be separable from the right kidney at this level but is contiguous with the right psoas muscle. The inferior vena cava is displaced ventrally by the mass and the right kidney still has a very lateral position. You may wonder about the soft tissue mass in the left upper quadrant. Oral contrast medium proved it to be small bowel.

The dilemma at this point should be clear to you. The mass certainly could be a pancreatic pseudocyst but the CT is not pathognomonic in any sense. It could also be a psoas abscess or a necrotic tumor. After some debate, you decide that the high amylase level most certainly indicates pancreatic disease.

Mr. R. S. agrees to a trial of conservative therapy, and followup studies show regression of the mass. The amylase level also diminishes over time. You are satisfied with the diagnosis of traumatic pancreatic pseudocyst and try to get him to change his madcap lifestyle.

MR. J. McG.

Mr. J. McG. is a very stubborn man with intermittent gallbladder problems who has always refused either to take his medication regularly or to have his gallstones removed. This time when you see him, however, he is plainly frightened about his health and says you can remove his gallbladder if doing so will stop his back pain. You find his abdomen soft and nontender but feel an unmistakable mass in the left upper quadrant. Ultrasound is planned first and demonstrates a large mass in the left upper quadrant. The relationship of the mass to the pancreas and the aorta is obscured by bowel gas, so you order a CT scan. The sections shown are made after infusion of intravenous contrast material and some oral contrast medium have been given. What do you see on the first two sections?

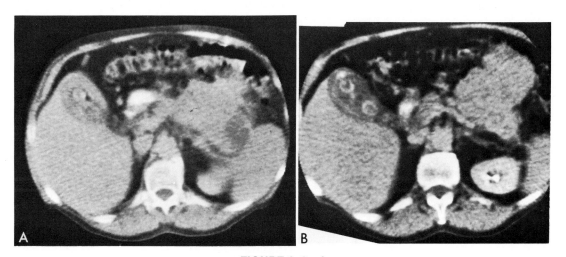

FIGURE 3–8a, b

There is a large irregular mass in the left upper quadrant that is displacing the splenic vessels dorsally. It is not homogeneous in attenuation and appears separate from the duodenum. The pancreatic head is not enlarged. While this mass should be your major interest, you could be forgiven for admiring the laminated gallstones that Mr. J. McG. has held onto for so long. The third section done about 6 cm below the others shows just how large this mass is.

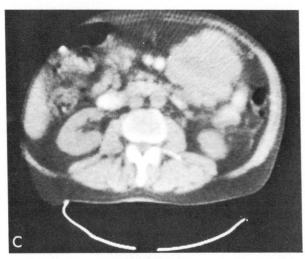

FIGURE 3–8c

You are certain that the patient has a carcinoma of the tail of his pancreas. His symptom of back pain is ominous but he is now anxious for surgery. Your diagnosis is confirmed when a bulky, partially necrotic tumor is removed. Though no obvious metastases are found at surgery, Mr. J. McG. does not fare well and dies about five months later.

It is important to stress that in this patient normal fat planes are maintained even though symptoms suggested that he had retroperitoneal spread of the carcinoma. Effacement of the fat planes is a better sign when present than when absent and is nonspecific in any case.

MR. P. G.

Mr. P. G., a 60 year old man, has been under your care for many years. He now complains of mid-epigastric pain and weight loss. An enlarged supraclavicular node is palpated and there is a vague suggestion of epigastric mass. A liver-spleen radionuclide scan is obtained after a biopsy of the supraclavicular node reveals metastatic adenocarcinoma. Is it abnormal?

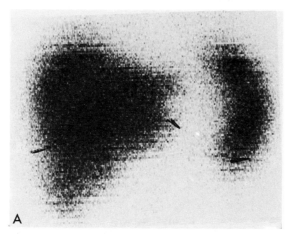

FIGURE 3–9a

This scan was obtained to evaluate the liver for metastases. The only defect is a notch in the left lateral margin of the left lobe. Though the notch could be an anatomic variant, metastases could have this appearance.

Upper gastrointestinal series, small bowel series and barium enema are all normal, as is chest radiograph. You order a CT scan to reevaluate the liver and to examine the pancreas and retroperitoneum. The initial section is shown below. Intravenous contrast medium has been given. What information is obtained?

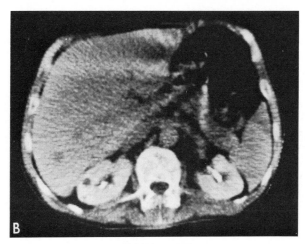

FIGURE 3–9b

Both kidneys are enhanced by contrast medium. The right kidney has two small round areas of diminished attenuation. These are small renal cysts. The renal veins are well seen, the left passing over the aorta and beneath the superior mesenteric artery to join the inferior vena cava. The tail of the pancreas is seen behind the stomach, in a normal relation to the left kidney and the spleen. The liver is not homogeneous. Much of this appearance is due to bowel gas artifact but in the right lobe there are two small vague round areas of decreased attenuation. In the left lobe just medial to the stomach there is a larger area of diminished attenuation. This is in the area of questionable abnormality on the radionuclide scan and is clearly abnormal, though the artifacts make it hard to see well. The most likely explanation is metastasis. What do you make of the next section, 2 cm more caudal?

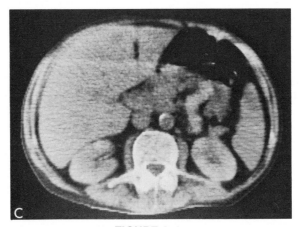

FIGURE 3–9c

The liver is again abnormal with several poorly defined areas of diminished attenuation; the most obvious ones are anterior in the right lobe and near the junction of the caudate lobe and the right lobe. The striking finding is the lobulated mass in the body of the pancreas anterior to the aorta. Does the next section add any more information?

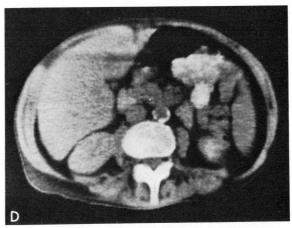

FIGURE 3–9d

The head of the pancreas is normal. The descending duodenum is filled with very dilute contrast material. Anterior and to the left of the aorta there is a lobulated soft tissue density that is paraaortic adenopathy. There is another area of diminished attenuation in the liver, unfortunately traversed by an artifact.

These scans show a mass in the body of the pancreas with metastases to liver and paraaortic nodes. The patient refuses a percutaneous guided needle aspiration of the mass and is placed on chemotherapy. A postmortem examination eight months later confirms the pancreatic carcinoma.

While radionuclide scanning is the primary method for evaluating the liver for metastases, CT scanning can be valuable in cases in which the findings are equivocal. CT scanning also has the advantage of examining adjacent organs at the same time.

CASE 3–10:

MRS. L. B.

Mrs. L. B. is a 65 year old woman who has no use for doctors and has been well all her life. She has had increasing jaundice and pruritus for the last four months however and now has developed epigastric pain. Her family finally forces her to seek medical aid. Physical examination discloses an icteric woman with a firm, somewhat enlarged liver. Below the liver there is an epigastric fullness. Her serum chemistries are those of severe obstructive jaundice. In view of the clinical findings, an ultrasound scan is ordered and it demonstrates dilated intrahepatic ducts. Because the mid-abdomen is obscured by gas, a CT scan is ordered to evaluate the pancreas. The first section was done just below the tip of the xyphoid. Oral contrast material has been given. What do you see?

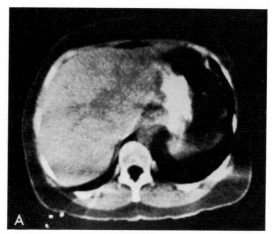

FIGURE 3–10a

There is a stellate low density radiating from the hilum of the liver. This pattern can be caused by either dilated portal veins or a dilated biliary system. Intravenous contrast medium is often needed to make the differentiation without a clinical history, but since the biliary system is known to be dilated in Mrs. L. B., it is not necessary. The next section is 6 cm lower. What do you see?

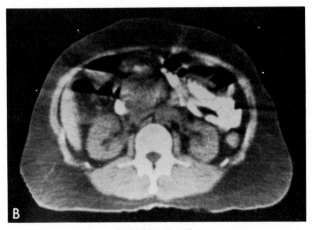

FIGURE 3-10b

The gas in the transverse colon is the cause of the difficulty that the ultrasonographer encountered. On the CT scan the bowel gas has caused some artifact but usable information still can be obtained. A 5 cm mass present in the head of the pancreas displaces the adjacent bowel. Posterior to the mass the normal fat plane between the pancreas and the inferior vena cava is not seen. This is a somewhat difficult distinction to make on a scan plagued with artifacts, but the other retroperitoneal fat planes are preserved. The CT diagnosis is a carcinoma of the pancreatic head with spread into the peripancreatic fat. These findings are confirmed at surgery and the patient is treated with biliary and gastrointestinal bypass.

This case illustrates the ability of CT to obtain pancreatic images when ultrasound is technically impossible. It also illustrates that these methods can be used together in the successful diagnosis of pancreatic disease.

CASE 3–11:

MRS. L. C.

One of your patients with poorly controlled diabetes, Mrs. L. C., comes in because of abdominal distention and episodes of vomiting during the last several days. Her urine sugar is 4+ and her blood glucose over 700 mg%, so you hospitalize her. Abdominal films show a markedly distended stomach; a nasogastric tube is placed for decompression. Copious amounts of fluid and food are removed. When her diabetes is under control, the nasogastric tube is removed so that a gastrointestinal series can be performed but, overnight, the vomiting returns. You also learn that her bilirubin is now slightly elevated. You decide that a CT scan of the upper abdomen will most efficiently provide the information you need; you have one performed that morning.

Four scans are illustrated, which cover about 12 cm of the patient's abdomen. You need to look at all four to reach a primary diagnosis. There are several related abnormalities and at least one incidental finding. What are your observations?

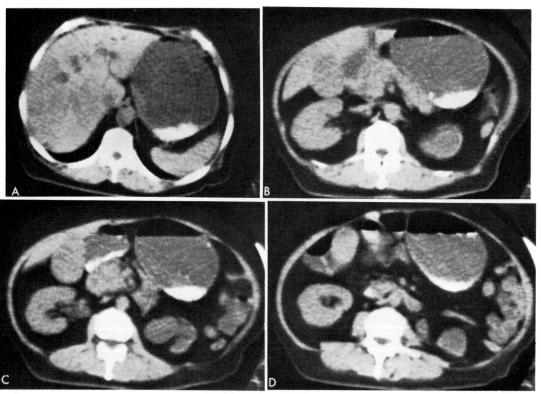

FIGURE 3–11a, b, c, d

The most obvious abnormality on all four sections is the markedly dilated stomach. It is filled with fluid and the Gastrografin has layered in the dependent portions of the stomach. On section c in particular you should observe the unusually ventral position of the antrum. In fact, the antrum is draped over a soft tissue mass, a portion of which is duodenum with some fluid. The remainder is the pancreatic head. Section b also shows the antrum draped over the mass, though no Gastrografin is present. The body and tail of the pancreas are seen on section b and are normal but the gallbladder is large. In fact, you also see it on sections c and d. When you check section a, central lucencies suggest dilated bile ducts. At this point you should feel confident in saying that Mrs. L. C. has a mass in the head of the pancreas, most likely a carcinoma, which is causing both gastric outlet obstruction and extrahepatic biliary obstruction. The tumor has not obscured the fat planes dorsal to the pancreas but the gastric outlet obstruction indicates that a cure is unlikely. Surgery is required to relieve Mrs. L. C.'s jaundice and gastric outlet obstruction however and a final decision can be made then.

Did you make the incidental observation? The left kidney is small and has very little parenchyma remaining. It seems to be a small hydronephrotic sac with a large extrarenal pelvis, which is seen in scan c.

Amazingly, Mrs. L. C. tolerates surgery well, but your findings are confirmed. She has always wanted to see the Taj Mahal in the moonlight, so after promising to take proper care of her diabetes, Mrs. L. C. goes to India with her husband.

CASE 3–12:

MRS. E. M.

Mrs. E. M., a 66 year old retired school teacher, returns to your office complaining of abdominal pain. Eight months ago she was seen with similar complaints and an extensive workup at that time resulted in a cholecystectomy for chronic cholecystitis. On physical examination now an upper abdominal mass seems to be present, and she mentions a weight loss of ten pounds. You decide to request a CT scan. The initial section is through the upper abdomen. Intravenous and oral contrast material have been given. What structures are seen and are they normal?

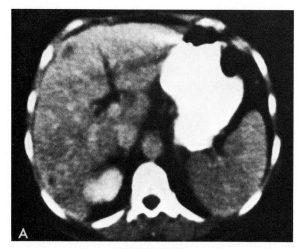

FIGURE 3–12a

The liver, the spleen and the upper pole of the right kidney are seen. The stomach is distended with contrast medium. Portal veins are opacified and fat is radiating from the hilum of the liver. In addition, there are two small irregular areas of diminished attenuation in the periphery of the liver. The spleen is somewhat enlarged. What do you make of the next section?

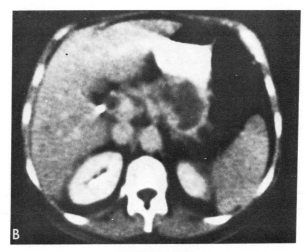

FIGURE 3–12b

There are more small areas of diminished attenuation in the liver and the spleen is large. The most striking abnormality is seen behind the stomach. There is a large irregular area of diminished attenuation in the body and tail of the pancreas with a thick irregular wall. Is the next section helpful?

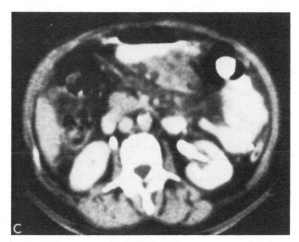

FIGURE 3–12c

The head of the pancreas is normal. The superior mesenteric artery and vein are seen anterior to the aorta. Posterior to the antrum this scan shows further evidence of the mottled mass. What do you see on the final section?

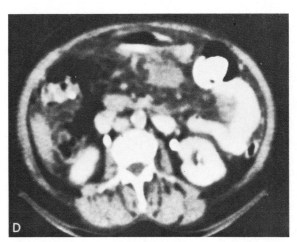

FIGURE 3–12d

The mass is extending into the mesentery. If you review sections *b*, *c*, and *d* together, you can say with some assurance that the mass arises in the body and tail of the pancreas and has grown into the mesentery by direct extension. The low density areas in the liver are metastatic foci, and the splenic enlargement results from obstruction of the splenic vein. The large area of low attenuation in the mass is probably necrotic tumor, though a cystadenocarcinoma is a less likely possibility. Clearly, resection for cure is not possible.

At surgery a large necrotic carcinoma of the pancreas is found and hepatic metastases are confirmed. The unfortunate Mrs. E. M. has a rapid downhill course and dies in two months.

Your patient Mr. J. R. has just had a long and difficult cholecystectomy and common duct exploration. Now, three days after surgery, he has severe abdominal pain, a high fever, an increasingly high white blood cell count and progressive hypotension. You suspect a retained common duct stone and ascending cholangitis with gram-negative sepsis. An emergency T-tube cholangiogram is done that changes your worries dramatically. What is demonstrated?

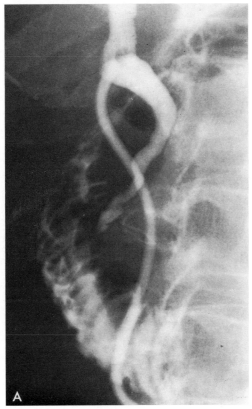

FIGURE 3–13a

There is free flow of contrast material into the duodenum and no stones are seen; however, the duodenum is markedly abnormal. The sweep is widened and its folds are thickened and spiculated. These findings suggest an inflammatory process in the pancreas. An emergency serum amylase shows marked elevation. An ultrasound evaluation of the pancreas is limited by bowel gas, but the ultrasonographer tells you that the pancreas is diffusely enlarged and appears to have areas of diminished echogenicity compatible with edema or fluid collections. A CT scan is suggested to try to better evaluate the pancreas. The initial section illustrated is at the level of the origin of the superior mesenteric artery. Oral and intravenous contrast material have been given. What information is obtained?

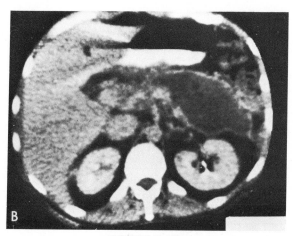

FIGURE 3–13b

The distal body and tail of the pancreas are markedly enlarged, and only a thin rim of tissue remains surrounding a large area of mottled, diminished attenuation in the tail. Fat planes are preserved. The next section illustrated is about 2 cm caudad to the first. What is seen?

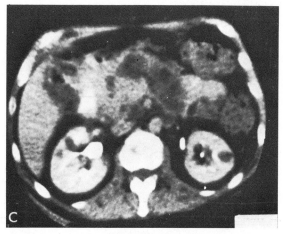

FIGURE 3–13c

The head and proximal body of the pancreas are also enlarged and contain irregular areas of mottled low density. In light of the clinical picture, the extensive diffuse abnormality of the pancreas is most compatible with acute postoperative pancreatitis with autonecrosis and abscess formation. You should have also noticed several small areas of decreased attenuation in the kidneys, which are small cysts.

Because of continued deterioration of his condition, Mr. J. R. is returned to the operating room and the CT findings are confirmed at laparotomy. Multiple drains are placed and he has a long and complicated convalescence.

The clinical history is the only grounds on which this CT scan can be correctly interpreted. Pancreatitis with pseudocysts or carcinoma of the pancreatic head obstructing the pancreatic duct could both have this appearance on CT scans.

MRS. H. G.

Mrs. H. G. is a charming older woman who has been your patient for many years. She has a bad back and does exercises for her stomach muscles daily. She has just come home from a cruise to the Galapagos Islands, however, and her cabin was too small for exercises. Now she is exercising extra hard to make up for the two week hiatus. She comes in complaining of abdominal pain. While you suspect that her pain is muscular, you request an ultrasound examination to exclude any intraabdominal pathology. Mrs. H. G. did have a breast carcinoma removed about six years ago and she is concerned about recurrence of her cancer. You are quite surprised, however, when the ultrasonographer calls to say that he has found a mass in the tail of the pancreas.

A single transverse section of the ultrasound which shows the mass is illustrated. What are your thoughts about the mass?

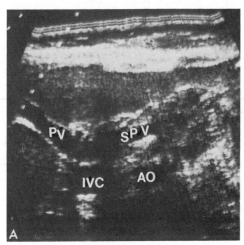

FIGURE 3–14a

The portal vein (PV) and splenic vein (SPV) are well seen. Normal pancreas is seen ventral to the splenic vein. The left lobe of the liver lies beneath the anterior abdominal wall. The inferior vena cava (IVC) and aorta (AO) are labelled. To the left of the splenic vein and aorta is a round mass, which is clearly separate from the liver. It has a rather coarse echo pattern; although it transmits sound rather well, the contents are not fluid. These two factors lead the ultrasonographer to suggest that the mass may not be the usual pancreatic adenocarcinoma.

Mrs. H. G. has become asymptomatic now and you cannot feel a mass. An upper gastrointestinal series is normal except for an extrinsic posterior impression on the body of the stomach. After discussing the dilemma with Mrs. H. G. and her surgeon, you decide to request a CT scan to characterize the mass more completely.

Four sections from the CT study are demonstrated. Two are done before intravenous contrast medium is given and two are done after. The levels are similar. You should look at all four sections, identifying the pancreas and the mass, and then try to characterize the mass. Does it appear similar to the pancreatic carcinomas you have already seen?

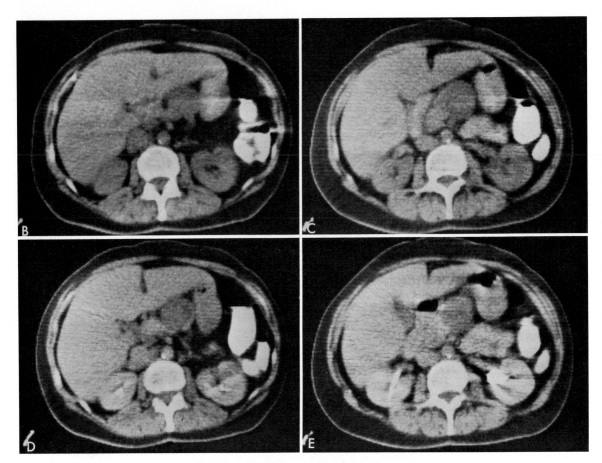

FIGURE 3–14b, c, d, e

Scans *b* and *c* demonstrate the mass lying ventral to the aorta and superior mesenteric artery and dorsal to the left lobe of the liver. It clearly arises within the pancreas. An atrophic pancreatic tail is seen on *b*, extending posterolaterally from the mass. The fascinating observations you make when comparing *b* and *c* to *d* and *e* are that there is rim enhancement in the mass and it is generally lower in CT density than the remainder of the pancreas after contrast medium has been given. Both observations differ from those in the usual CT picture of pancreatic adenocarcinoma.

A careful review of the entire CT scan demonstrates no additional abnormalities. The patient decides to have an exploratory laparotomy. The surgeon reports that the lesion looks just as it did on the two scans. It is found to be a <u>cystadenoma</u>. Mrs. H. G. does well postoperatively and goes off to Mazatlan to recuperate.

A word of caution is in order. CT experience with cystadenomas and cystadenocarcinomas is very limited and we cannot say how often the findings seen here will occur. It would seem unlikely that CT scanning will be able to differentiate between benign and malignant forms of cystadenoma in the pancreas, though the findings of distant spread or extension into adjacent structures would answer this question. Certainly, the rim enhancement of the mass by contrast material is not common with pancreatic carcinomas and should suggest the possibility of another type of lesion when it is observed. <u>Rim enhancement is not specific for neoplastic lesions and may be seen in inflammatory lesions.</u>

KIDNEY AND ADRENAL
CT SCANNING

Computerized tomography is an adjunct to the evaluation of the kidneys by intravenous urography and ultrasound. The renal parenchyma and collecting systems are well seen both with and without the use of intravenous contrast material at CT scanning. Intravenous urography is the primary radiographic technique for evaluation of the collecting systems, for detection of renal masses and for determinaiton of renal function.

The distinction between cystic and solid renal lesions can be made rapidly by ultrasound in most patients. If the results of sonography are inconclusive or the examination cannot be performed for technical reasons, CT can be used to evaluate the nature of a mass. Generally, CT of the kidneys should be reserved for more complex situations such as evaluating the extrarenal extent of a known renal carcinoma. CT can be used to identify fat within a renal mass and to confirm the diagnosis of angiomyolipoma. CT does not supply detailed information about the vascular anatomy of the kidney, though some information about the main renal artery and vein and the inferior vena cava can be obtained. It is not a replacement for angiography in the evaluation of solid renal masses or in other situations in which detailed information about renal vascular anatomy is important.

Since CT very graphically displays the kidney and the surrounding structures, it is an excellent means of assessing perirenal pathology such as hematoma, abscess and urinoma. The transaxial view of the kidney is also an excellent means of assessing that organ for focal parenchymal loss. Areas of acute vascular compromise can be delineated with the use of intravenous contrast material. Hydronephrosis may be demonstrated, especially if the collecting structures are at least moderately distended. CT has a place in screening patients with acute onset of renal failure if obstruction cannot be demonstrated by other means.

Two points should be quite clear at this juncture. First, CT rarely has a primary role to play in the evaluation of the kidneys. Other simpler, less expensive tests give as much information about the kidneys as renal CT scanning does. Second, almost every CT scan of the abdomen will include the kidneys in part or completely, and much can be learned about the kidneys with this technique.

The adrenal glands also lie in the retroperitoneum adjacent to the upper poles of the kidneys. No very good radiographic screening examination exists for the adrenal glands. Plain films of the abdomen may show very large adrenal masses or adrenal calcifications and an intravenous urogram sometimes shows renal displacement or axis deviation by a moderate-sized adrenal mass. Ultrasound can demonstrate some adrenal masses, but these must be relatively large lesions that can be cleared from the ribs before they are detectable. Adrenal venography cannot be classed as a screening test, since it has definable morbidity and is technically somewhat difficult to perform consistently. It can, however, demonstrate masses as small as 5 or 6 mm. Radionuclide scans can be performed, but these are not generally available and are expensive. This means that in carefully selected patients, CT scanning has a role in detection of malignant or benign tumors and possibly in adrenal hyperplasia.

The adrenal glands are routinely seen at CT scanning if the patient has enough body fat to separate the glands from larger adjacent structures. Diffuse enlargement and masses of 2 cm or more can be seen fairly regularly. Adrenal configuration is variable, so subtle changes must be interpreted with care.

NORMAL KIDNEYS AND VARIATIONS

CT scans of the kidneys make transverse sections through the organ to produce an image that is very different from the standard radiograph. The kidneys are positioned lateral to the spine and rarely extend anteriorly to the middle of the abdomen. The right kidney lies caudad to the left in most patients. Generally, scans made every two centimeters for six cuts starting two to four centimeters below the xyphoid tip will include both kidneys. However, the examination should be modified to conform to individual variations in anatomy as information is obtained during the study.

The kidneys generally need evaluation both before and after injection of intravenous contrast material. The volume of contrast medium need not be large, though when visualization of the ureters is important, a larger infusion will help.

The CT scans that follow are from several patients with normal kidneys. You should identify all the major structures on each scan and notice the variations in renal position, shape and size. Also observe the relative attenuation of the kidneys compared to other organs.

The first section is at about 4 cm below the xyphoid. What do you see?

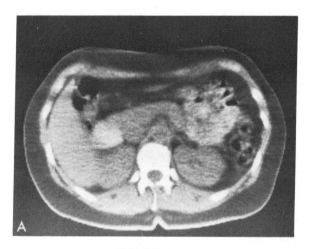

FIGURE 4-1a

The right lobe of the liver occupies the right lateral abdomen and medial to it next to the spine is the upper pole of the right kidney. The duodenum is immediately ventral to the kidney and the body of the pancreas is anterior to the aorta. The section crosses the left kidney in the upper portion of the collecting system so that some peripelvic fat is seen centrally. It is difficult to distinguish the inferior vena cava from the pancreas. Small bowel loops are filled with contrast material.

The next two sections were performed 4 and 6 cm below the xyphoid in another patient. Try to identify blood vessels in particular.

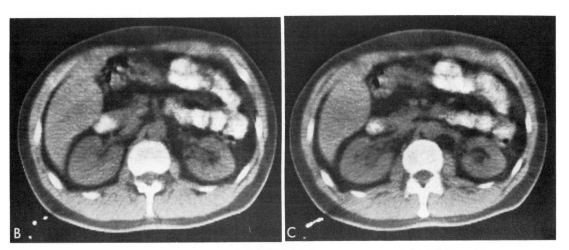

FIGURE 4–1b, c

Renal arteries and veins are generally seen if the appropriate sections are obtained. In this patient the scans are clearly in mid-kidney bilaterally, though slightly lower on the left than on the right. On scan *b* the superior mesenteric artery is originating from the aorta and the inferior vena cava is seen to the right of the aorta. A blood vessel is entering the right renal hilum. It does not seem to enter the inferior vena cava; therefore, it is probably the right renal artery. On *c* the left renal artery arises laterally from the aorta but leaves the plane of the section before reaching the kidney. The right renal vein is seen entering the inferior vena cava. When the left renal vein can be seen in scans, it generally crosses anterior to the aorta below the superior mesenteric artery. The superior mesenteric artery and vein are seen on end in *c* just ventral to the duodenum.

You should also notice the distribution of renal parenchyma, which is thicker laterally than medially. The kidneys have a slightly lower attenuation than the liver.

The next two sections are made before and after injection of intravenous contrast material. What do you see?

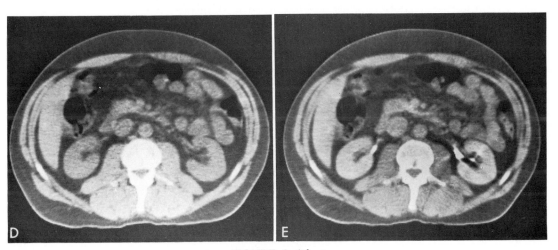

FIGURE 4–1d, e

The scans were done through the middle of the kidneys. The right lobe of the liver is seen on the right and many bowel loops are seen. The inferior vena cava is rounded and larger than the aorta, which suggests that this patient performed a Valsalva maneuver during both scans. On scan *e* the collecting systems contain contrast medium. The peripelvic fat is still seen. On the left, the very dense contrast material is causing an artifact. Using both scans, you can separate the left renal pelvis from a vessel immediately ventral to it. You cannot say whether this is renal artery or vein on this section, since the vessel leaves the plane of the cut before it can be identified.

The next two sections of two different patients were done in midabdomen following intravenous contrast medium injection. What do you see?

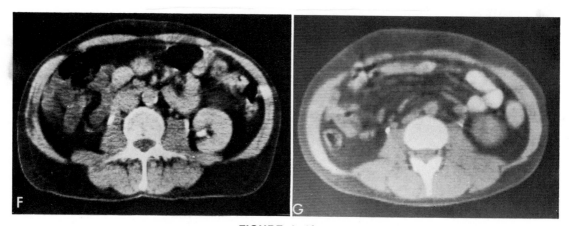

FIGURE 4–1f, g

In both patients, the right kidney is not in the plane of the section. The tip of the left kidney is seen in *g*, whereas the lower collecting system is seen in *f*. Both sections are shown to illustrate the usual position of the ureters lateral to the anterior border of the psoas muscles. While ureters can sometimes be distinguished without contrast medium, their opacification makes this identification much simpler.

Notice how flat the inferior vena cava is on *g*, and how round it is on *f*.

Developmental variations in kidney size, shape and position are rather common. These are usually well defined at urography but may be incidental findings at CT scanning. The kidney also can be affected by extrinsic masses that alter both its shape and position. What do you see on the next section?

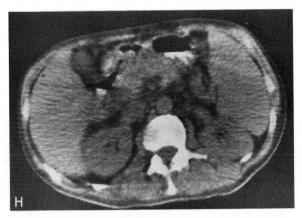

FIGURE 4-1h

The large spleen is compressing the left kidney medially and obscuring the fat planes around the kidney. In other situations, the kidney can be displaced ventrally or in a cephalocaudad direction.

MR. H. W.

Mr. H. W. is a 49 year old man who is undergoing staging for a non-Hodgkin's lymphoma. He had a positive supraclavicular node biopsy about two weeks ago and is referred to you because the right ureter is deviated medially on an intravenous urogram. The referring physician wants you to do a CT scan for retroperitoneal adenopathy. You review the intravenous urogram. What is your opinion?

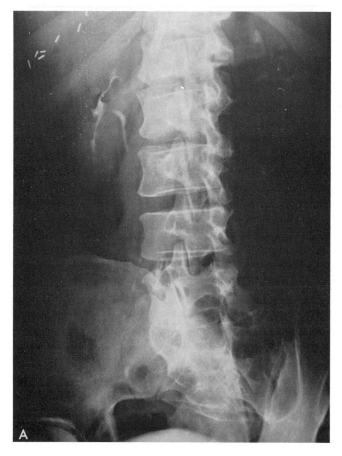

FIGURE 4–2a

Overall, the right ureter has a more medial course than is usual and on the right posterior oblique film, which is illustrated, you see multiple impressions on the ureter that make you suspect adenopathy.

CT scans were performed both before and after the infusion of intravenous contrast material. Oral contrast medium had also been given on the second set of scans. The scans illustrated were done at similar levels. You should be looking for an anatomical variation relevant to the patient's problem.

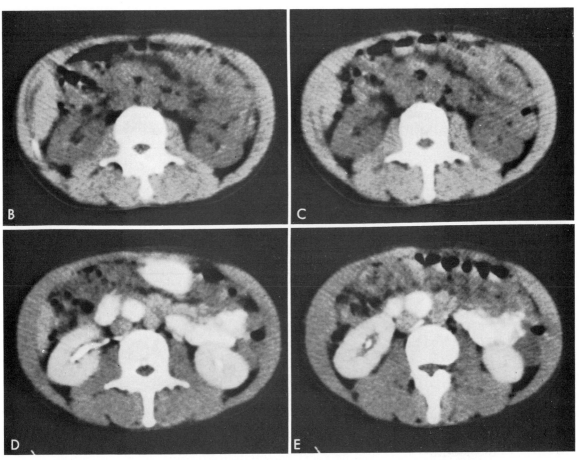

FIGURE 4-2b, c, d, e

Sections *b* and *c* are baseline scans that should help with your interpretation of sections *d* and *e*. The levels are not absolutely identical, but it is often not possible to obtain an exact match. The patient is thin; this makes the fat planes difficult to see. The important observations on *b* and *c* are negative ones: there are no enlarged lymph nodes and no masses.

Following administration of intravenous contrast material, the kidneys are densely opacified and the collecting systems are filled. The unusual course of the right ureter is the observation you should make. You notice that it lies behind the inferior vena cava. Retrocaval ureter is a developmental anomaly that is generally of no clinical significance, though it is sometimes associated with partial ureteric obstruction and the associated complications of hydronephrosis. In general, the frontal film of the urogram will show a characteristic medial course of the ureter, but in patients who may have retroperitoneal disease other studies are sometimes necessary to confirm the diagnosis.

As for Mr. H. W., he has no evidence of lymphoma beyond the original biopsy site. After radiation therapy, he does well and is free of clinically apparent disease.

CASE 4–3:

MR. Y. B.

Mr. Y. B., a 70 year old man with carcinoma of the bladder, returns to his doctor because of the gradual onset of left leg edema. It has been about 18 months since his radiation therapy and nephrostomy for hydronephrosis. Pelvic recurrence of the carcinoma is suspected and a CT scan is obtained to evaluate its extent. The initial scan is through the pubic symphysis. Is there any abnormality? Use your imagination, since the scanning of the pelvis is not discussed until later in this book.

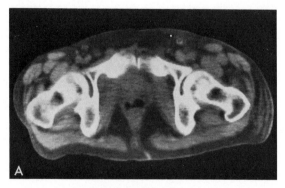

FIGURE 4–3a

There is mild enlargement of the prostate seen directly behind the pubic symphysis. The pelvic fat planes are normal and no mass is present. There is slight generalized enlargement of the muscles in the left groin.

What about the next level, 2 cm above the pubic symphysis?

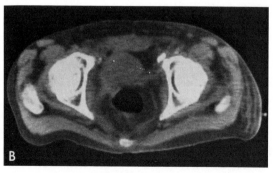

FIGURE 4–3b

The bladder is seen and is asymmetric, but no mass is displacing it. Some irregularity of the fat planes can be seen adjacent to the pelvic side walls, probably due to surgery and radiation therapy. No cause of unilateral leg edema is detected.

Scans were also obtained through the mid-portion of the kidneys. What are the major findings here?

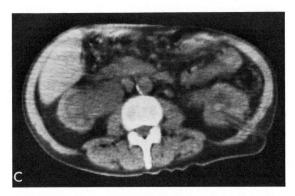

FIGURE 4-3c

The right kidney has a thin rim of cortex, which surrounds a massively dilated renal pelvis. The extrarenal pelvis extends medially and is actually displacing the inferior vena cava medially and ventrally. A percutaneous nephrostomy tube, which is in place in the left renal pelvis, can be seen traversing the skin and subcutaneous fat as well as the renal cortex to enter the renal pelvis.

The typical findings of hydronephrosis are well seen on the right. CT scanning can be used to differentiate acute renal obstruction from other causes of anuria when intravenous urography is not practical.

You are encouraged by the absence of pelvic masses; a venogram is performed. Extensive internal iliac and common femoral thrombophlebitis is demonstrated, which responds well to anticoagulation therapy.

CASE 4–4:

MRS. A. C. AND MR. W. G.

Mrs. A. C. and Mr. W. G. have nothing in common except that you request an intravenous urogram on both patients before each is to undergo pelvic surgery. Mrs. A. C. needs a hysterectomy for endometrial carcinoma, and Mr. W. G. has an enlarged prostate. In both patients, a small misshapen kidney is reported and there is also some concern about a mass lesion. Ultrasound is unsuccessful in Mr. W. G. and demonstrates a left renal cyst in Mrs. A. C. Her right kidney, the one of concern, is not well seen. You request renal CT scans on both patients.

Review a urographic film on Mrs. A. C. first. What are your concerns?

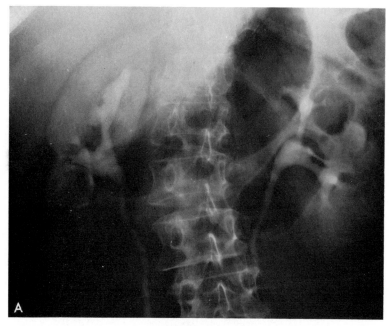

FIGURE 4–4a

There is spreading of the calyces in the mid-portion of the left kidney, which is the location of the renal cyst seen at ultrasound. On the right the lower pole is shrunken and a prominent scar is present along the lateral margin of the kidney. Some lower pole infundibulae are stretched, suggesting a mass.

A CT section done without contrast material is shown next. What does it show?

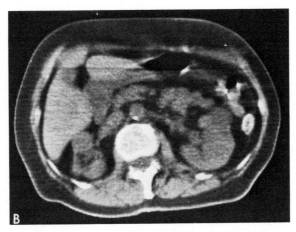

FIGURE 4–4b

The section is done at the level of the right renal scar and shows much more dramatically how much parenchymal wasting has occurred. The left kidney is enlarged by two slightly low density masses that you think are renal cysts. A scan enhanced by contrast medium at this level confirms this.

What additional information is available on a lower scan done after contrast medium infusion?

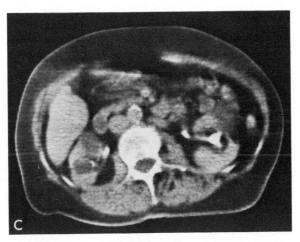

FIGURE 4–4c

The ventral left renal cyst is still seen peripherally. On the right the parenchymal wasting is less marked, and there are two small cysts to explain the calyceal displacement seen on the urogram.

Reassured about Mrs. A. C., you turn to Mr. W. G. and review his intravenous urogram. What do you see on the tomogram on the next page?

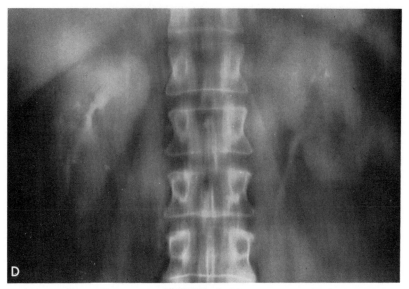

FIGURE 4–4d

The left kidney is small and has an irregular contour. One dominant bulge is seen on the lower pole laterally. You had hoped that ultrasound would define this mass better, but because ribs interfered, you have requested a CT scan. A single scan done after contrast medium is shown. What do you think now?

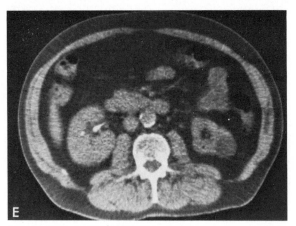

FIGURE 4–4e

The parenchymal thinning on the left is contrasted with the normal right kidney. This is a diffuse loss. A low attenuation lesion is seen laterally, which is not changed with contrast medium infusion. It is a simple renal cyst.

Both patients' cases illustrate the ability of CT scanning to demonstrate renal scarring and atrophy. This information is generally obtained by urography, but on occasion CT scanning can more completely define this type of defect. Renal cysts are well demonstrated by CT scanning and will be discussed in greater detail later in this chapter.

Mrs T. Q. is a 72 year old woman who has had a left renal calculus for many years. She has always been asymptomatic, but when she arrives in your office with severe back spasms and left costovertebral tenderness you suspect trouble and order an intravenous urogram. Two films are illustrated. What do you see?

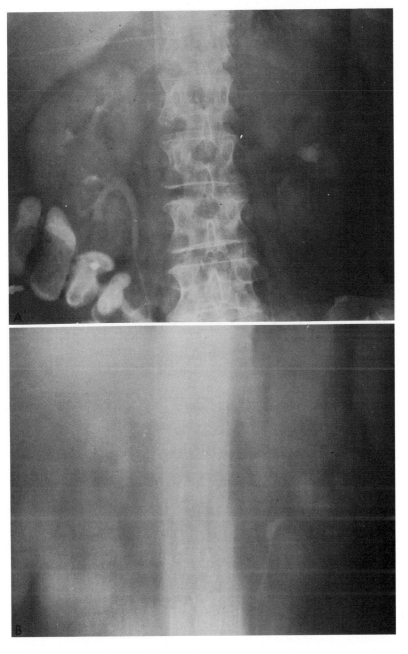

FIGURE 4–5a, b

The five minute film shows a normal right kidney. The renal calculus is superimposed over the left renal pelvis and the calyces are quite attenuated. The entire kidney appears bulbous and the upper pole is poorly defined. Tomograms done shortly after the five minute film also do not adequately demonstrate the upper pole. The calculus is not seen on this mid-kidney cut. These findings could be due to pyelonephritis but Mrs. T. Q.'s back spasms seem too severe. You wonder if she has a perinephric abscess and request an ultrasound. A longitudinal section from the ultrasound is illustrated and it increases your concern. What do you learn?

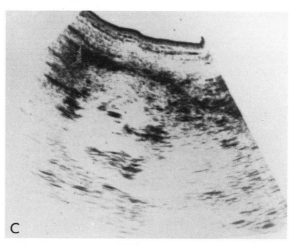

FIGURE 4–5c

The patient is prone. Dorsal to the kidney there is an amorphous soft tissue mass with a very transonic region that could be fluid. This collection corresponds to the area in which you could not see the kidney contour on the urogram. Clinically, an abscess is most likely and drainage will probably be necessary. You order a CT scan to get a better idea of the complete extent of the lesion. Three sections are illustrated. What do you see on the first one?

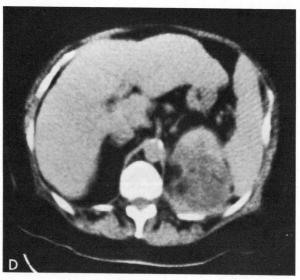

FIGURE 4–5d

The spleen is enlarged. More important, the upper pole of the left kidney is enlarged and has a mottled appearance. The lower attenuation regions are quite intimately involved with the more normal-appearing areas. You are somewhat surprised by the next section, about 8 cm lower. What do you make of it?

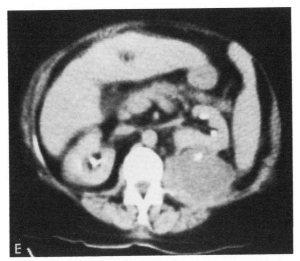

FIGURE 4-5e

At this level the left kidney is displaced ventrally but appears intrinsically normal. There is a large, low density mass dorsal to the kidney in the posterior perirenal space which contains the renal calculus Mrs. T. Q. has had so long. The mass is intimately related to the left psoas muscle. The final section, 4 cm caudad, is also interesting. What does it show?

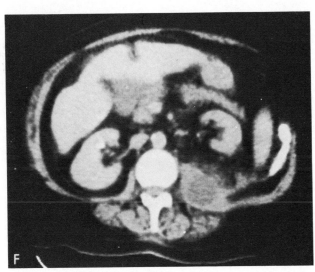

FIGURE 4-5f

The left kidney is still displaced but is surrounded by normal fat. The left psoas muscle is markedly enlarged compared to the right and has a central low attenuation area. The transversalis fascia on the left is markedly thickened when compared to the right. This fascia delineates the posterior perirenal space.

You now have a good idea what Mrs. T. Q.'s problem is. You believe that the renal calculus has eroded through the kidney into the dorsal perirenal space where the abscess began. The abscess involves the upper pole of the kidney but spares the remainder. Symptoms probably began when the abscess burrowed into the left psoas muscle, causing severe back spasms.

Mrs. T. Q. is started on antibiotic therapy, and the abscess is surgically drained. After a large collection of purulent material is removed, the back spasms diminish rapidly. After a slow but uneventful convalescence, Mrs. T. Q. returns home.

CASE 4–6:

MR. M. L. AND MR. R. C.

Mr. M. L. is a 64 year old gentleman you have known for years. He says that he has a reduced urinary stream and some vague right flank pain. You examine him and find an enlarged prostate, so he is admitted to the hospital for a urologic evaluation and possible cystoscopy. A single tomographic section of the intravenous urogram is illustrated. Do you see any abnormality?

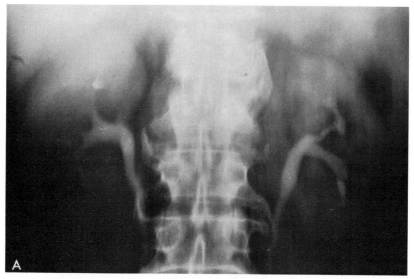

FIGURE 4–6a

The left kidney is normal, but on the right there is a lucency in the midportion of the kidney. You discuss this finding with the radiologist, who thinks that the lucency probably is a renal cyst. What test would you perform next?

Together, you and the radiologist decide to perform an ultrasound examination of the kidney, since in most cases this study will distinguish between a fluid-filled cyst and a solid mass. Later that afternoon, however, the radiologist calls to tell you that while the mass is most likely a cyst, he is not absolutely certain because of overlying rib artifact. He suggests a CT examination. The first section shown has been done prior to the administration of intravenous contrast material. Do you see the mass?

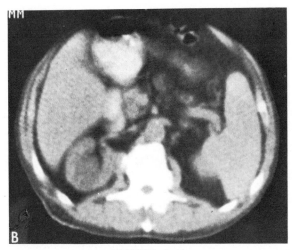

FIGURE 4–6b

In the midportion of the right kidney an ovoid area of decreased attenuation is present that corresponds to the mass seen on the urogram. The next section was obtained at the same level after intravenous contrast material had been given. What information is added?

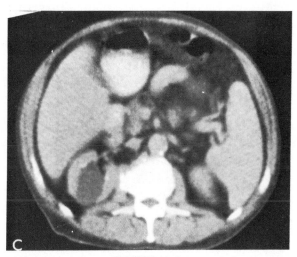

FIGURE 4–6c

The abnormal area in the right kidney now stands out in bold relief from the remainder of the kidney. The normal renal parenchyma has taken up the infused contrast material and has an increased x-ray attenuation. The abnormal area does not take up any contrast material from the blood stream and its attenuating ability remains unchanged. The measured CT number in the mass is 2, which is quite close to that of water. The mass is sharply defined and has very thin walls. Thus the mass shows all the CT features of a simple renal cyst.

That evening when you see Mr. L. on your rounds you learn that he is very much concerned about all the tests he has had. When told of the cyst, he becomes convinced that he has cancer and nothing you can say reassures him. The urologist has little luck in this regard and it is decided to aspirate the cyst. On aspiration 20 cc of clear fluid is removed. The cytologic examination of the fluid as well as the air and water soluble contrast material examination of the cyst are normal.

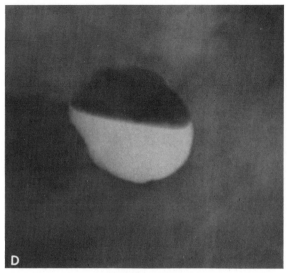

FIGURE 4–6d

Reassured, Mr. M. L. has his prostatism attended to and later presents the radiologist with a case of champagne as a token of gratitude.

Your disconcerting experience with Mr. M. L.. — a large amount of trouble over a small cyst — reminds you of Mr. R. C., in whose case the reverse is true. Mr. R. C. is a middle aged patient with widespread malignant melanoma. A CT scan was performed to aid in therapy planning. The radiologist brings over the dramatic section illustrated below. What do you think of this renal mass?

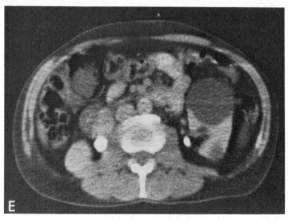

FIGURE 4–6e

The radiologist has brought only a scan done after infusion. A very large mass is seen arising from the anterolateral aspect of the left kidney. The interface between the mass and the kidney is very sharp, and at its margins there are "beak-like" extensions of normal renal tissue embracing the mass. The attenuation in the mass is low compared to the renal parenchyma. The radiologist tells you it measured 3 and did not change with the contrast infusion. The wall is very thin. This mass has the CT characteristics of a large simple renal cyst. You should note that there is a second area of abnormality dorsally. This is the upper portion of another cyst better seen on lower sections.

Mr. R. C. cares nothing about his renal cysts and wants only to get on with his chemotherapy, which has postponed a marriage to a young lady about half his age.

Mr. E. T. has a prostate carcinoma and an abdominal CT scan is ordered to help stage his disease. No adenopathy is seen, but sections through his right kidney are not normal. What do you see on the section done before contrast medium was infused?

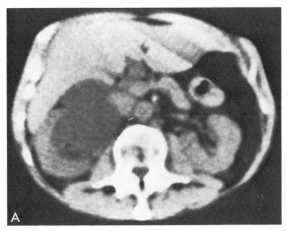

FIGURE 4–7a

There is a large, somewhat lobulated, low density area in the medial aspect of the right kidney. The right renal parenchyma looks thinner than that on the left. It is tempting to think that this low density structure is a large renal cyst, but are you sure?

The next scan is at about the same level but dilute oral contrast medium and intravenous contrast medium have been given. What observation can now be made about the right kidney?

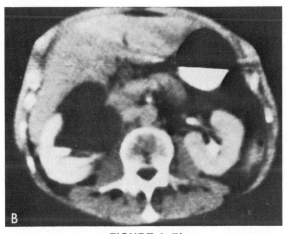

FIGURE 4–7b

The renal parenchyma has been markedly enhanced by the intravenous contrast medium and contrast medium is being excreted bilaterally. The appearance on the left is normal. On the right there are several fluid levels between opacified urine and the fluid in the large low density structure; this structure can thus be identified as a dilated renal pelvis. The final section is about 6 cm caudad. It confirms your diagnosis.

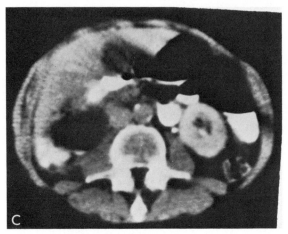

FIGURE 4–7c

There is a normal-sized, nonopacified right ureter immediately medial to the dilated renal pelvis. It lies between the right psoas muscle and the inferior vena cava in a position similar to that of the opacified left ureter. This is a difficult observation, but one that can be made. Review of the entire study helps in making this decision. At this point you should be quite confident that you are dealing with a ureteropelvic junction obstruction. You get a film of the abdomen following the CT scan.

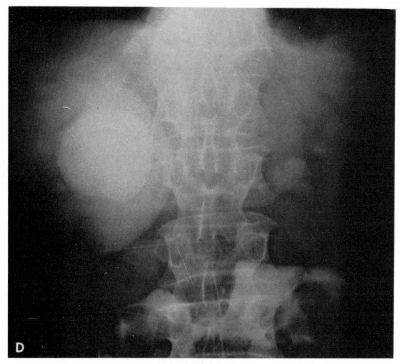

FIGURE 4–7d

The oral contrast medium is now in the colon. A normal left renal collecting system is faintly seen. On the right the dilated renal pelvis and calyces are classical for ureteropelvic junction obstruction.

Mr. A. S. is a 79 year old man who had a transurethral prostatectomy about eight years ago. At that time an intravenous urogram demonstrated bilateral renal cysts. There were several small cysts on the right and a single large left one. Over the past year he has been having increasing difficulty with urination; now he comes in with hematuria. Intravenous urography is done even though you expect to find no change in his kidneys and in fact have scheduled the patient for cystoscopy.

The situation changes when the radiologist calls and says that he has found a new mass, which is probably solid, at the left lower pole. Ultrasound of the kidney confirms the presence of solid mass and also raises the question of retroperitoneal tumor spread, so you request a CT scan. No adenopathy is seen, but the scans done both before and after contrast material infusion demonstrate clearly the differences in CT appearance of cysts and solid masses. What do you see on the first two sections?

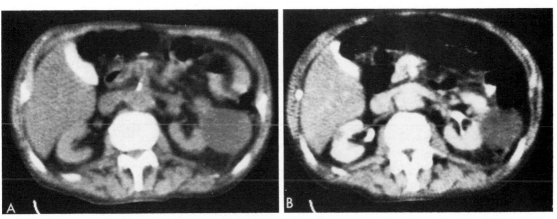

FIGURE 4–8a, b

These sections demonstrate the left renal cyst before and after infusion of contrast medium. On *a*, the cyst is rounded and has a lower attenuation than the renal parenchyma. The separation between the cyst and the normal parenchyma is quite distinct. After the contrast medium infusion, the distinction is even sharper. The attenuation number of the cyst has not changed. Notice the small right renal cyst, which was not seen before the contrast medium, and also notice the enhancement of arteries and veins. Contrast these figures with the next two.

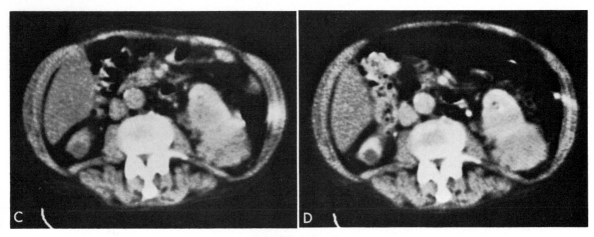

FIGURE 4–8c, d

These sections are made about 6 cm distal to the first pair. A small right renal cyst is seen on both sections. The left kidney now has a bulbous deformity of the lower pole that is irregular in contour, nonhomogeneous in attenuation and poorly separated from normal kidney. With infusion of contrast material, the mass becomes slightly more distinct from the normal kidney, but its attenuation also increases somewhat. These findings are typical of a solid mass.

Needless to say, these distinctions are often less clear-cut. Multiple cysts and small cysts may be confusing, as may a highly necrotic tumor. The differences between renal cysts and solid renal masses seen here do form the basis of the diagnostic decision process.

Mr. A. S. has no evidence of distant spread of his renal cell carcinoma and does well after nephrectomy. Recently he brought in his first great grandchild for you to admire.

Mr. J. F. comes to see you because of hematuria and flank pain. He also complains of weight loss and a low grade fever. Physical examination is unrevealing and you decide to do an intravenous urogram. What do you see on the film that is illustrated?

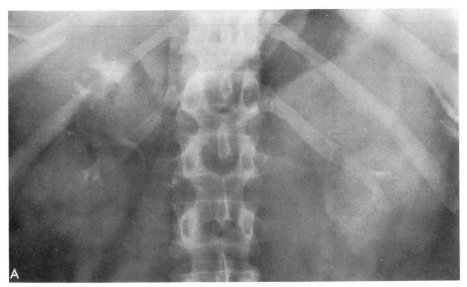

FIGURE 4–9a

The left renal contour is well seen at the lower pole but is obscured superiorly. The axis of the left kidney is different from the axis on the right and the lower pole is displaced laterally. An ultrasound examination reveals a large solid mass arising from the left upper pole. Because of the size of the mass, a CT scan is requested to more fully define the extent of disease before angiography. What do you see in the first section done at the diaphragm?

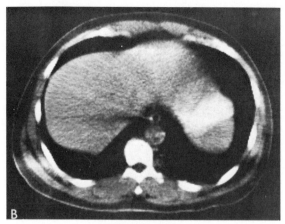

FIGURE 4–9b

The abnormality at this level is a small area of increased attenuation behind the left diaphragm just behind the descending aorta. This is an enlarged posterior mediastinal lymph node. There is air in the esophagus.

What about the next section? Intravenous and oral contrast material have been given.

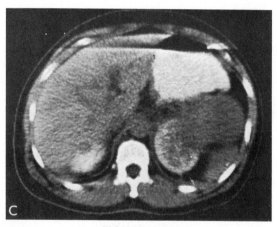

FIGURE 4–9c

A large mass extends laterally from the left kidney. The spleen has a dense calcification, probably an old granuloma. You should notice that part of the left kidney has been replaced by tissue that does not take up contrast medium normally. Does the next section add any information?

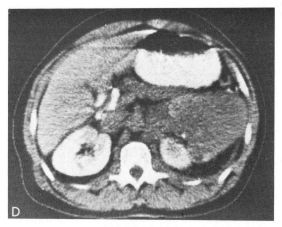

FIGURE 4–9d

Here the mass is even larger, extending to the lateral abdominal wall. There is another bulky mass in the left renal hilum, and the aorta is displaced anteriorly and to the right. The tail of the pancreas is elevated and seems thinned.

The next scan also has a striking abnormality. What do you think of it ?

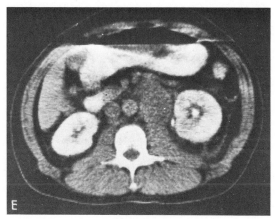

FIGURE 4–9e

A large paraaortic mass obscures the left psoas, displacing the aorta to the right. The inferior aspect of this paraaortic mass extends along the psoas muscle dorsal to the kidney. This mass explains the confusing axis deviation seen on the intravenous urogram. What do you see on the final section?

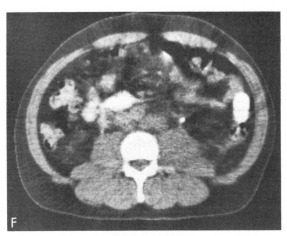

FIGURE 4–9f

The fourth portion of the duodenum is displaced ventrally and the aorta to the right by the mass. At this level the paraaortic nodes are enlarged and the mass involves the left psoas muscle diffusely.

Clearly, extensive metastatic disease involves the mediastinal and paraaortic nodes and the left psoas muscle. The renal hilum is enlarged, suggesting renal venous obstruction. This is confirmed at angiography.

The sheer bulk and extent of the tumor is quite discouraging, but a palliative resection is undertaken using an anterior surgical approach. The surgeon confirms most of the CT findings, though he does not attempt to do a complete nodal exploration. Pathological diagnosis is renal cell carcinoma.

Mr. J. F. thinks about his rather unfavorable prognosis while convalescing and decides to give chemotherapy a chance.

Mr. F. G. is a 74 year old man whom you first saw several months ago for microscopic hematuria. At that time a right renal cell carcinoma was diagnosed that proved to be unresectable at surgery. He has been doing rather well since discharge, but now comes to your office with peripheral edema. You suspect that the tumor must be compressing the inferior vena cava or growing into it and suggest inferior vena cavography to prove this. Mr. F. G., reluctant to have another vascular study, asks if anything else could be done. You decide to try a CT scan. The first two sections demonstrated were done in the upper abdomen before and after intravenous contrast material had been infused. What unusual observation can you make?

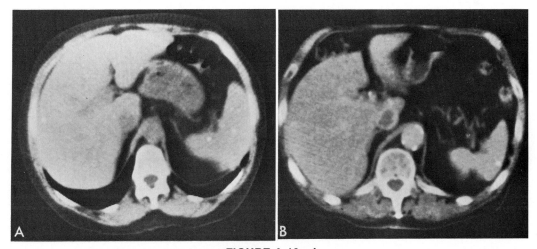

FIGURE 4–10a, b

Aside from a small splenic calcification scan *a* shows no definable abnormalities and should be used only for comparison with *b*. The striking finding on this section is the intraluminal filling defect in the inferior vena cava as it enters the liver. The filling defect has an irregular contour, and you are sure it is caused by renal cell carcinoma growing into the inferior vena cava. Normal portal veins are faintly opacified.

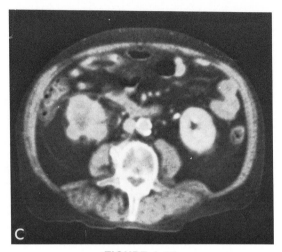

FIGURE 4–10c

Figure 4–10c is a section through the primary renal tumor. It clearly is not adjacent to the inferior vena cava and so cannot be causing peripheral edema by direct compression. It has a very irregular contour and a low density center, suggesting necrosis.

After much debate, arterial infarction is decided upon with the hope of diminishing tumor bulk. The preinfarction angiogram shows a typical renal cell carcinoma with some arteriovenous shunting into the inferior vena cava and tumor growing into the inferior vena cava.

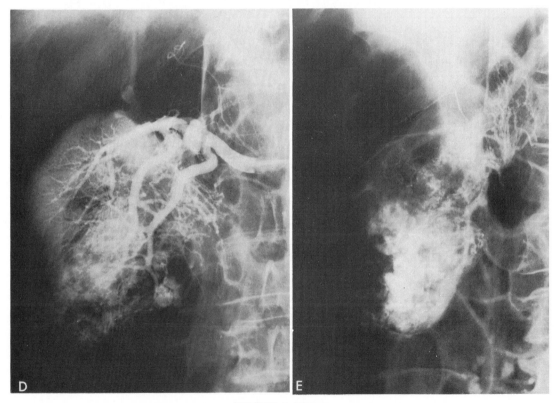

FIGURE 4–10d, e

Mr. F. G. has several days of pain after the infarction but when he begins to recover from the infarction procedure, his peripheral edema is diminishing.

Mr. D. L. is a 45 year old man who had a lung resection four months ago for carcinoma. He has not done at all well since surgery, and you readmit him to the hospital because of dehydration, severe back pain and depression. A bone scan does not demonstrate the expected bony metastases so you order an intravenous urogram, suspecting his pain to be renal in origin. The study is limited by patient motion and diminished renal function but suggests bilateral masses.

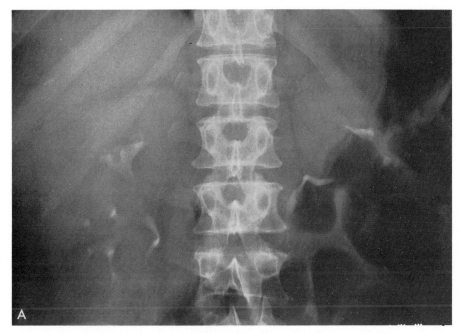

FIGURE 4–11a

The patient refuses to lie prone for an ultrasound examination and in desperation you request a CT scan. Mr. D. L. tries to cooperate but cannot hold his breath for the entire scanning period so the study is not completely satisfactory. It does answer your questions, however. Two sections performed after injection of intravenous contrast medium are illustrated. What do you see on the first?

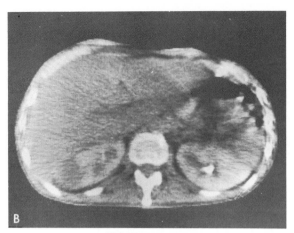

FIGURE 4–11b

The upper section shows at least two low density lesions in the right kidney. These are relatively poorly defined and are of higher density than the usual renal cysts. The left kidney appears bulky on this scan. Look at the lower scan now.

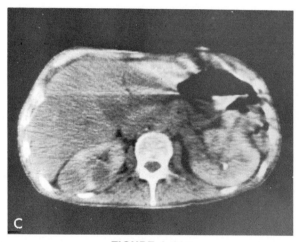

FIGURE 4–11c

The second section also shows the right renal lesions. On the left a mass is seen arising from the ventral lateral surface. What do you think these moderately low density lesions are?

The patient refuses any further therapy and dies two days later. An autopsy reveals bilateral renal metastases from the lung carcinoma. Though renal metastases from lung carcinoma are found rather frequently at autopsy, it is quite unusual to encounter metastases large enough to detect clinically. The CT picture of renal metastases is that of any solid renal tumor.

NORMAL ADRENALS

The adrenal glands generally lie adjacent to the upper poles of the kidneys bilaterally. The right adrenal gland is seen adjacent to the liver, usually lying in a notch created by the junction of the right and the caudate lobes. This space is bounded medially by the right crus of the diaphragm. The left adrenal gland is often seen in the retroperitoneal fat dorsal to the pancreatic tail and the splenic vein, to the left of the superior mesenteric artery and the aorta and ventral and medial to the tip of the left kidney. Both glands can have a three-pointed or triangular shape, though the right is often rather linear. Use of intravenous contrast medium may aid in the evaluation of adrenal masses, especially larger ones. Oral contrast medium is not usually needed when evaluation of the adrenal glands is the sole purpose of the CT scan.

Each of the next five scans illustrated was taken on a different patient. Locate the adrenal glands on each scan but also identify the rest of the structures. You should be aware again of the many variations of the human abdomen. What do you see on the first section?

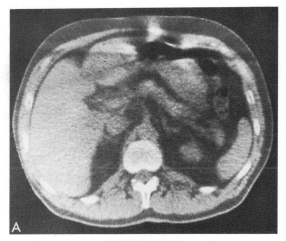

FIGURE 4–12a

This scan demonstrates the splenic tip, the body of the pancreas anterior to the origin of the superior mesenteric artery, both the right and left lobes of the liver and the upper pole of the left kidney as well as both adrenal glands. The left adrenal gland is the triangular structure lying beside the aorta and superior mesenteric artery dorsal to the pancreas. The right adrenal gland lies immediately dorsal to the inferior vena cava. It would be more fully seen on a scan done about 1 cm cephalad to this one. What is on the next scan?

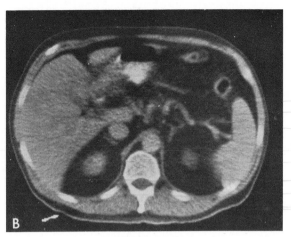

FIGURE 4–12b

Perhaps the most striking finding on this section is the splenic vein running from the splenic hilum toward the midline. Lying in the fat bordered by the left kidney, the aorta and the splenic vein is the left adrenal gland, which has a three-pointed configuration. The right adrenal gland is immediately dorsal to the inferior vena cava. The top of the right kidney is also seen. The gastric antrum contains some contrast material, and the right lobe of the liver is seen. What do you see in the next patient?

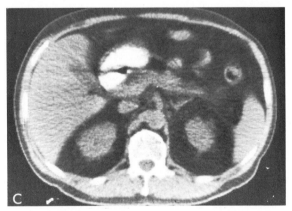

FIGURE 4–12c

Here both kidneys, the spleen, the right hepatic lobe and both the gastric antrum and duodenum are demonstrated. The body of the pancreas is anterior to the superior mesenteric artery. To the left of the superior mesenteric artery dorsal to the pancreatic tail is the left adrenal, which is quite triangular. Two normal nodes are just medial to the left adrenal gland. Do you see the right adrenal gland?

The right adrenal gland in this patient was seen on sections 2 and 4 cm cephalad but is not demonstrated at this level. How about the next scan?

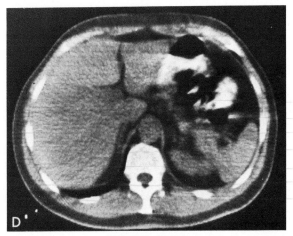

FIGURE 4–12d

This scan is dominated by the right and left lobes of the liver. Stomach, spleen, colon and left kidney are also seen. A portion of the left adrenal gland is demonstrated ventral to the kidney, but other sections display it better. The right adrenal gland is between the diaphragm and the right lobe of the liver and is linear in appearance. What do you see in the final patient?

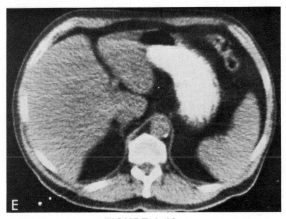

FIGURE 4–12e

The liver, spleen and stomach are the primary organs demonstrated. The right adrenal gland is comma shaped and lies in the bed of fat between the diaphragm and the inferior vena cava. The left adrenal gland is not seen on this section.

It should be apparent that both adrenal glands vary in configuration and location. Since the glands are quite small, scanning at 1 cm intervals is reasonable once each gland is located. Even closer sectioning may be indicated in specific cases, particularly when small lesions such as adenomas producing endocrinopathy are being sought.

MRS. B. L.

Mrs. B. L. is a 36 year old woman who comes to see you complaining of an increase in body hair and especially the development of a beard. She does indeed have many stigmata of a virilizing syndrome. On physical examination, she is moderately obese and has dark striae on her abdomen. In addition, you feel a left upper quadrant mass that prompts you to order an intravenous urogram. In the interval between her visit to you and the intravenous urogram, she has some left flank pain. What do you see on the tomographic cut that is illustrated?

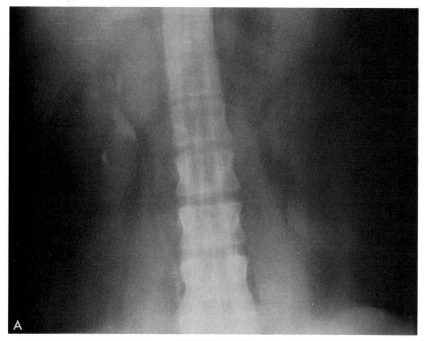

FIGURE 4–13a

The right kidney is normal in size and function. The left kidney lies much lower than the right — a somewhat unusual relationship — and is quite bulky. No collecting structures are seen. There is a suggestion of increased soft tissue in the left upper quadrant but no definite mass is seen. The remainder of the intravenous urogram shows delayed function on the left without evidence of obstruction of the collecting system.

It seems probable that Mrs. B. L. has an adrenal tumor causing virilization and also the unusual position of the left kidney. You can't readily explain the change in left renal function, however. You order a CT scan to try to confirm your thoughts about an adrenal tumor and to examine the left kidney. The CT scan is performed the day after the intravenous urogram. There is residual contrast medium in the left kidney. Four sections from the CT scan are shown. What observation can you make on the first section?

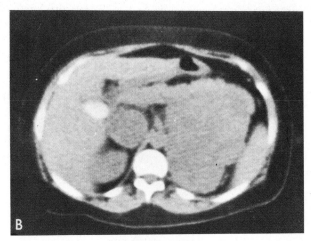

FIGURE 4–13b

A very large soft tissue mass fills much of the left abdomen at this level. The mass obscures the diaphragm medially and may actually involve it. The aorta and the superior mesenteric artery are normal. The inferior vena cava is markedly enlarged. The pancreas is separated from the mass by a very thin fat plane but is displaced ventrally by the mass and the inferior vena cava. Contrast medium is seen in the gallbladder. Since no gallbladder contrast medium has been given, this must be due to vicarious excretion of the urographic agent given the previous day. The next section illustrated is performed 6 cm below the first. What do you see?

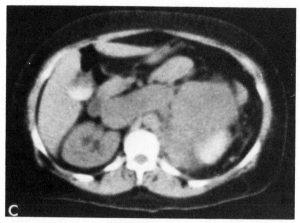

FIGURE 4–13c

The mass is smaller at this level and an area of higher density is present peripherally. You suspect that this is the upper pole of the left kidney, since you know it still contains contrast material. The right kidney is normal and is not opacified. A large tubular structure crosses anterior to the aorta to join the inferior vena cava. You know it is not the pancreas and it does not look like duodenum. What are your thoughts about this structure and does the next section, 4 cm caudad, help?

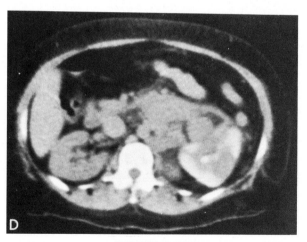

FIGURE 4–13d

The mass is even smaller at this level and the striking findings involve the left kidney. A very abnormal patchy nephrogram is seen on this and the next section. Round soft tissue masses are present adjacent to the aorta and dorsal to the kidney. In the renal hilum, there is an additional round mass of the same diameter as the tubular structure seen in c. This is the dilated left renal vein filled with tumor and the patchy nephrogram is probably caused by venous infarctions of the kidney. The final section, Figure 4–13e shows the nephrographic defects better and also shows adenopathy.

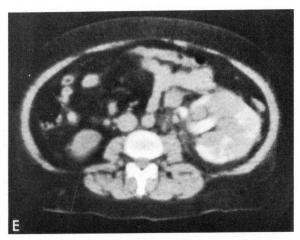

FIGURE 4–13e

You believe that you have demonstrated a very large left adrenal neoplasm that is displacing the pancreas and the left kidney. It has involved the left renal vein and the inferior vena cava, causing venous infarcts of the left kidney. It has spread to retroperitoneal lymph nodes and you think it may involve the diaphragm.

You talk over the situation with the surgeon and Mrs. B. L. The magnitude of the tumor makes resection very difficult. The patient, however, requests that the surgeon try, since chemotherapy may be aided by "debulking." This procedure proves very difficult, but the surgeon does resect the major portion of the tumor. Mrs. B. L. has a massive pulmonary embolus shortly after surgery and dies. Surgery and autopsy confirm your findings.

This case emphasizes the efficiency of CT scanning in assessing the extent of a mass without an extensive invasive procedure such as angiography.

CASE 4–14:

MR. L. A.

Mr. L. A. is a 68 year old man who sees his doctor because of weight loss and cough. He has smoked cigarettes for 50 years. Though he has chronic bronchitis and brings up copious sputum in the morning, he has felt well and has not wanted to stop smoking despite repeated requests from physicians and family. Six months ago, however, his cough increased and became blood streaked. He began to feel weak and lose weight. Fearing the worst, he deferred medical consultation but now his doctor has ordered PA and lateral chest films. What do these show?

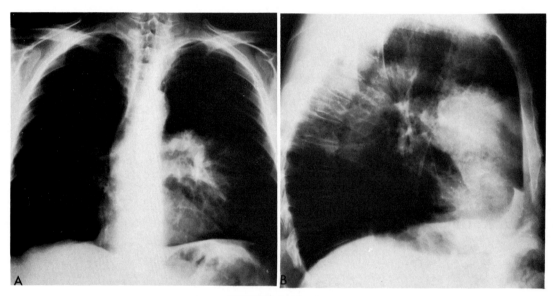

FIGURE 4–14a, b

There is a large mass lesion adjacent to the left hilum with associated consolidation of the lingula. Bronchoscopic examination and cytology confirm the clinical diagnosis of bronchogenic carcinoma. The tumor is found to be unresectable and a CT scan is obtained to help in planning the radiation therapy. What normal and abnormal structures can you identify on the section illustrated?

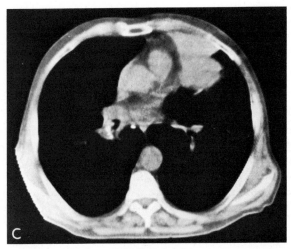

FIGURE 4–14c

The scan has been carried out through the mass below the level of the carina. The descending aorta is anterior to the spine to the left of the midline. The thin linear structure just anterior to the descending aorta is the pleural interface between the two lungs. In the anterior mediastinum, the left atrium and the aortic outflow tract are well seen. Anterior and to the left of the aortic outflow tract is the pulmonary outflow tract. These structures are surrounded by normal epicardial and pericardial fat. Just to the left of the mediastinum and inseparable from it is the pulmonary mass lesion, oval in shape. Beyond the mass is the consolidated lingula, occupying the anterior cardiothoracic sulcus.

After radiation therapy, Mr. L. A. feels better and does not return to you for eight months. He then comes in with pain in the left upper abdomen and the back. Since you fear metastases to bone, a bone scan is performed, which is negative. A supine film of the abdomen is then obtained. There is a subtle abnormality that you should try to detect.

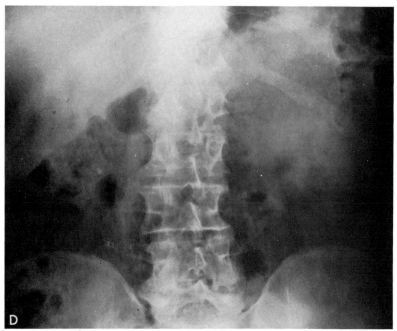

FIGURE 4–14d

The left renal axis is slightly altered with some rotation of the left kidney. This finding, in addition to a sense of increased soft tissues in the left upper quadrant, suggests an adrenal mass. A CT scan is requested to evaluate the left upper quadrant. The initial scan is through the level of the fundus of the stomach, which is distended with dilute contrast medium. What structures do you see?

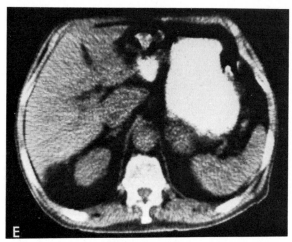

FIGURE 4–14e

The liver is in the right upper quadrant. The caudate lobe is rather prominent. There is a small triangular density just dorsal to the caudate lobe, surrounded by retroperitoneal fat. This is the normal right adrenal. Dorsal to the right lobe of the liver is the oval upper pole of the right kidney. Dorsal to the fundus of the stomach is the spleen against the posterior abdominal wall. The tortuous vessel passing into its hilum is probably the splenic artery. Medial to the spleen is another oval density. What is this? While it is tempting to call this density the upper pole of the left kidney, it is too medial and too ventral to be in the position the kidney would normally occupy.

The next section is 2 cm caudal to the first. What do you think of the findings?

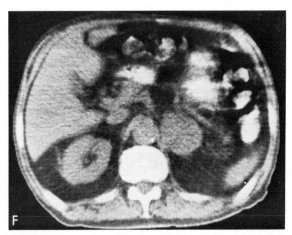

FIGURE 4–14f

The right kidney and its peripelvic fat are well seen. The oval density on the left is much larger, and the fat plane is compressed between it and the left crus of the diaphragm. Anterior to the mass is the splenic vein.

The next scan is 4 cm more caudad. What structures have now come into view?

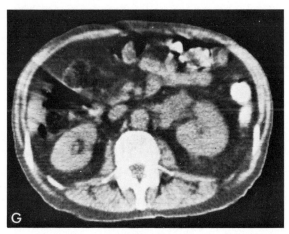

FIGURE 4–14g

The left kidney is seen lateral to the mass. This relationship should help you decide what the mass is. While the mass is intimately related to the kidney, it is always separated from it by a thin fat plane.

This mass is characteristic of an enlarged adrenal gland. It would be an improbable pattern of growth for either a primary renal tumor or a renal metastasis to the adrenal gland. In view of the clinical history, the adrenal mass is most likely a metastasis from the bronchogenic carcinoma. The upper abdominal pain is palliated with local radiotherapy.

CASE 4–15:

MR. G. B.

Mr. G. B., a 50 year old man, is referred for urologic evaluation because of a two month history of left flank pain and one episode of hematuria. An intravenous urogram is ordered. You are shown a single nephrotomogram. Is there anything of concern?

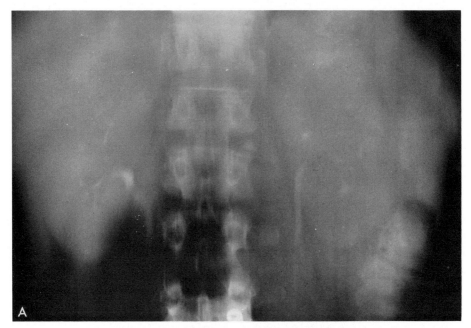

FIGURE 4–15a

The right kidney is normal. There is a mass involving the upper pole of the left kidney with effacement of the collecting structures and expansion of the upper pole. What study would you request next?

The most helpful simple study is an ultrasound to determine if the mass is a solid lesion or a deformity secondary to a renal cyst. A sonogram obtained in this case shows the lesion to be composed of solid tissue.

The next study requested by the consulting urologist is renal angiography. A late arterial phase film is demonstrated. What observations can you make?

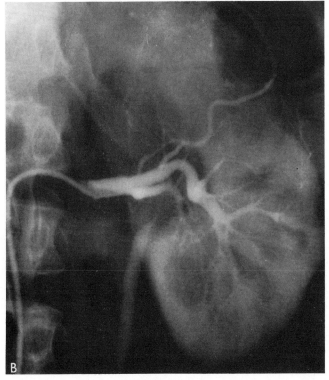

FIGURE 4-15b

The selective injection of the left renal artery shows a hypovascular mass in the left upper pole. There is encasement of an upper pole inter-segmental artery as well as the proximal portion of a large perforating capsular artery. Subtle fine neovascularity is seen extending into the mass.

The angiographer believes that the mass extends beyond the renal capsule, and a CT scan is obtained to determine the extent of the tumor. The initial section is at the level of the xyphoid. Since the scan was obtained soon after the angiogram, only post-contrast scans were obtained. What is your evaluation of the section on the next page?

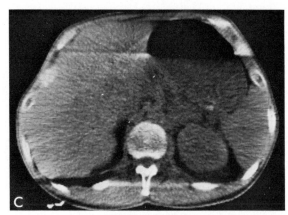

FIGURE 4–15c

The structures seen in the left abdomen include the stomach, which contains fluid and gas, and the wedge-shaped spleen. Dorsal to the stomach and to the left of the aorta is the left adrenal gland, which is enlarged and difficult to separate from adjacent structures. Behind the adrenal is the left upper pole renal mass. The renal capsule appears intact except anteriorly. There a tiny tongue of tissue seems to extend through the fat plane to the left adrenal.

The next section illustrated is through the left renal hilum. What further observations can be made?

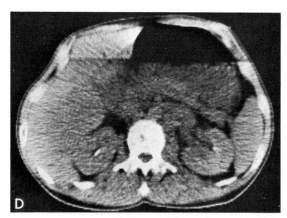

FIGURE 4–15d

At this level the left kidney is normal with a homogeneous enhancement by contrast medium. There is increased soft tissue between the left psoas muscle and the renal vessels. This is adenopathy in the renal hilum and paraaortic regions. The involvement of the left renal hilum and the left adrenal gland is confirmed at surgery, and a radical nephrectomy is performed for the renal cell carcinoma.

CT evaluation of renal neoplasms can accurately assess the extent of disease, particularly extension beyond the renal capsule and involvement of adjacent organs and lymph nodes. Extension into the renal vein is not consistently diagnosed by present CT techniques; therefore, angiography remains an important diagnostic procedure for many of these patients.

CT SCANNING IN THE RETROPERITONEUM

In the past, the radiographic evaluation of retroperitoneal disease has depended on indirect evidence acquired by opacification of structures such as the ureters or the inferior vena cava. Displacement or obstruction of these structures provides clues about the presence of disease.

The retroperitoneal lymphatic channels and lymph nodes may be visualized only through the use of pedal lymphography. Other methods developed to evaluate this area, such as retroperitoneal pneumography, have fallen into disuse because they produced significant morbidity. Ultrasound can provide considerable information about mass lesions involving the retroperitoneum and bulky retroperitoneal adenopathy may be defined. Evaluation of the retroperitoneum by ultrasound may be seriously limited by bowel gas.

CT provides excellent visualization of the tissue planes and structures of the retroperitoneum. The great vessels are well seen, and in patients with adequate fat, normal sized lymph nodes are seen. Adenopathy is recognized only when there is nodal enlargement since internal architecture of nodes cannot be evaluated by this method at present. One special advantage of CT is the ability to define the relationship of mass lesions to the vertebral bodies and to identify bony destruction. CT is able to demonstrate the retrocrural spaces and other hidden areas that are not seen by older methods.

Both oral and intravenous contrast material are useful in CT scanning of the retroperitoneum, but both must be appropriately used. Dilute oral contrast material should generally be used to distinguish bowel loops from retroperitoneal nodes and masses. The contrast material should be dilute enough so that it does not obscure small objects in the retroperitoneum or generate artifactual streaks. The oral contrast medium should be given at least 30 minutes before an examination if the lower retroperitoneum is in question. Contrast material or air can be given by rectum when needed to identify the distal large bowel, though this is not frequently needed.

Intravenous contrast material may be given for several reasons. When opacification of the vascular system is the prime concern, either a bolus injection or a bolus injection superimposed on an infusion should be used. Bolus injection should be made as near to the time of scanning as possible, and, in general, it will be necessary to do scans both before and after the administration of contrast material. In these patients it is very easy to exceed reasonable contrast medium dosages, so care must be taken when deciding what sections to make. Infusions of contrast material are generally used for organ enhancement and for improved definition of masses. Again, studies done both before and after contrast medium is given are generally indicated. When visualization of the ureters is of primary concern, a large volume infusion helps to insure continuous filling.

The information that can be obtained about the retroperitoneum using CT scanning is immense, but the technique should be judiciously used. Scanning intervals and the precise areas for scanning, which must be decided for each patient, depend on the reason for the examination and body habitus and ability of the patient to cooperate. Study of the retroperitoneum at 1 cm intervals is generally not necessary; it is very lengthy and tiring for most patients. The optimal study is one tailored to the situation at hand.

NORMAL RETROPERITONEUM AND VASCULAR STRUCTURES

The retroperitoneum has been included on every scan you have viewed thus far in this book, and you have already learned about the pancreas and kidneys, the most frequently studied organs of the retroperitoneum. This chapter emphasizes the other structures in the retroperitoneum — the blood vessels, the lymph nodes, the ureters, the muscles and other connective tissue. Many of these structures have been difficult to demonstrate in the past but CT demonstrates them well, facilitating the diagnosis of diseases involving this compartment of the body.

The retroperitoneum is variable from patient to patient. The cases illustrated emphasize this point and also demonstrate the various structures you can evaluate in the retroperitoneum. While you should try to identify all the structures on each section, devote the greater part of your attention to the retroperitoneum.

The first two scans were done 2 cm apart at the level of the second lumbar vertebral body. What do you see?

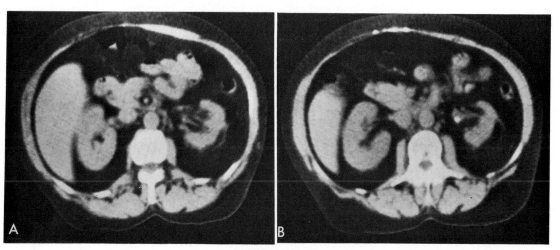

FIGURE 5–1a, b

The irregular, shrunken left kidney probably attracted your attention first. The patient has had multiple left renal calculi; a small one is seen in the renal pelvis. The aorta is almost in the midline and, especially on section b, many normal prevertebral lymph nodes are seen on both sides of it. The inferior vena cava is quite rounded and full, suggesting that the patient performed a Valsalva maneuver during both scans. On section b the right renal vein can be seen entering the inferior vena cava. The superior mesenteric artery, seen clearly on a, is surrounded by a halo of fat. To its right and slightly ventral is the superior mesenteric vein, which is difficult to see on this section. Contrast medium infusion would help in this identification. On section b the superior mesenteric vein is easier to identify.

You should have noticed the asymmetry of the psoas muscles. This degree of asymmetry may result from a variety of causes, such as improper patient positioning, scoliosis, an old cerebrovascular accident or poliomyelitis in childhood. Tumors or inflammation can cause the enlargement of one psoas muscle. Therefore, such findings must be interpreted with a good knowledge of the clinical history. In this patient, the asymmetry was due to a mild scoliosis. You will notice that the vertebral body is not quite straight in its anteroposterior orientation.

Some of the head of pancreas is seen, as is the tip of the liver and many fluid-filled loops of bowel. There is extensive retroperitoneal and intraperitoneal fat. Contrast these scans with a section at about the same level on another patient.

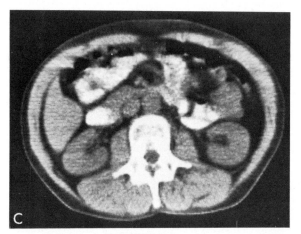

FIGURE 5–1c

This patient has much less fat than the first one. This is a 65 year old man, and the first patient was a 54 year old woman. As a rule, males have less fat than females of a similar habitus. The smaller amount of fat makes separation of the various structures much more difficult. In the emaciated patient, recognition of organ boundaries is often impossible.

The structures seen in this patient are the same as those in sections *a* and *b*, though the lymph nodes are less well seen. The psoas muscles have the usual degree of symmetry. The superior mesenteric artery and vein are seen just ventral to duodenum and pancreatic head. Some of the renal vasculature is demonstrated.

What do you see on the next section?

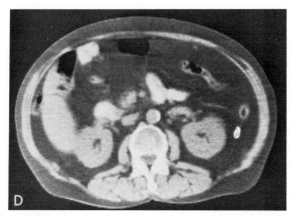

FIGURE 5–1d

This section was made slightly lower than the first three but both kidneys can be seen. The inferior vena cava is less distended, suggesting that this patient did not perform a Valsalva maneuver during the scan procedure. Dorsal to the inferior vena cava against the vertebral body is a semicircular soft tissue structure. This is in a common position for lymph nodes, but here it is the rounded end of a diaphragmatic ligament, which often has a very low attachment to the spine. Cuts done more cephalad show this structure to flatten out as it becomes more obviously part of the diaphragm.

What about the next section?

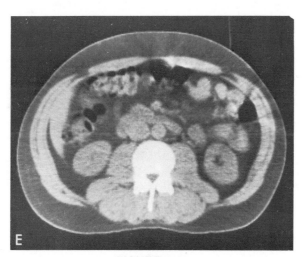

FIGURE 5–1e

This patient is a young man who is less fat and more muscular than any of the earlier patients. No oral contrast medium is present in the third portion of the duodenum, which is intimately related to the inferior vena cava. Although the two structures do have slightly differing attenuations, use of contrast material would make separation much simpler.

What do you see on the next scan?

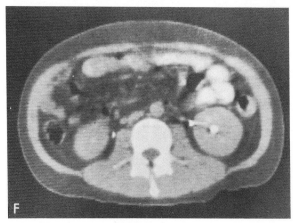

FIGURE 5–1f

Intravenous contrast material has been given and both ureters are seen adjacent to the psoas muscles. The position seen here is common but ureteric position is variable; the ureters often lie ventral to the psoas muscles, especially lower in the abdomen. They are not always symmetrical in position, though they often are. The inferior vena cava has a flat oval configuration on this section. Several lymph nodes are seen in the prevertebral area.

The next scan was made near the umbilicus. What do you see?

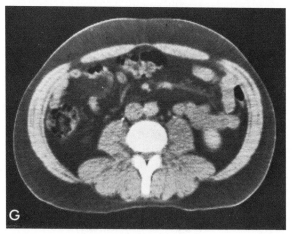

FIGURE 5–1g

Intravenous contrast medium has been given and the right ureter is opacified. The left ureter is not, but it can be seen in a similar position adjacent to the psoas muscle. When ureteric visualization is of primary interest, a large volume infusion of contrast medium will tend to fill the ureters steadily, assuring a good demonstration. However, densely opacified ureters will cause artifacts, so smaller amounts of contrast material should be used when possible. Lymph nodes are again seen and, incidentally, some mesenteric vessels are seen in the fat of this woman's mesentery.

The last section illustrated was made well below the umbilicus. What do you see here?

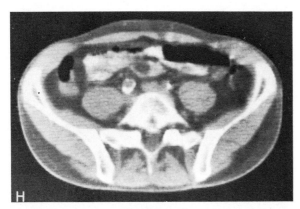

FIGURE 5–1h

The aorta has divided into the common iliac arteries, which can be identified by the calcification in their walls. The common iliac veins are seen together just to the right of the midline. The shape of the psoas muscles is rather round at this level. The iliacus muscles are seen along the iliac wings. Bowel occupies most of the section.

The normal retroperitoneum extends from the diaphragm to the true pelvis. The CT scan is uniquely able to aid in study of the retroperitoneal space and you should check this area on every scan you read. Because it is highly variable in appearance, only by repeatedly observing its configuration will you develop a sense of the range of normal and abnormal.

MR. J. D.

Mr. J. D. is a 28 year old gardener who has Hodgkin's disease diagnosed on cervical node biopsy. As part of his evaluation he has a pedal lymphogram, which is normal. Later he has an abdominal CT scan to evaluate areas not demonstrated by lymphography. Do you see any opacified nodes on these first sections?

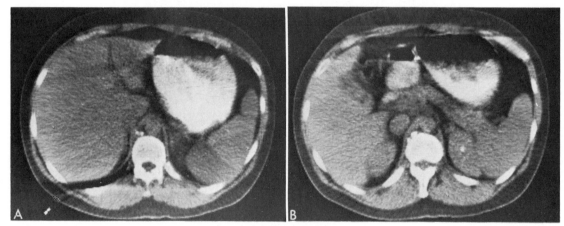

FIGURE 5–2a, b

These sections are from locations high in the abdomen, where nodal filling at lymphography is inconsistent. The small nodes seen behind the right crus of the diaphragm are normal retrocrural lymph nodes that are not usually opacified by pedal lymphography. Other lymph node-bearing areas at these levels are the celiac nodes and nodes in the hila of the spleen and liver. What do you see on the next sections?

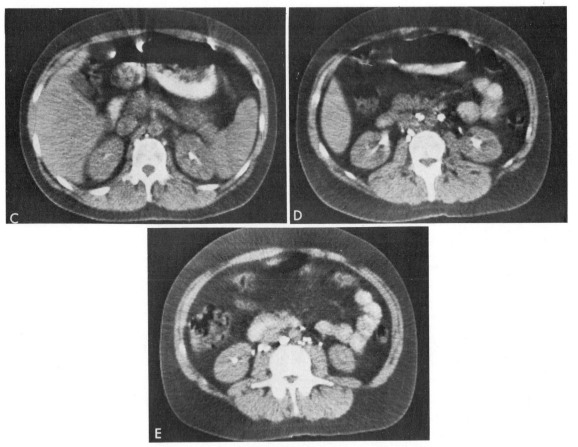

FIGURE 5-2c, d, e

On section *c* only retrocrural nodes are opacified. The section allows further evaluation of the hilum of the liver, the pancreatic bed and the hilum of the spleen, all of which are normal. The next two sections show normal opacified paraaortic and paracaval nodes at the level of the third portion of the duodenum. The mesenteric root is evaluated on these sections and no abnormal nodes are seen. Notice how the nodes surround the aorta and the inferior vena cava and drape over the anterior aspect of the psoas muscles. The next sections show nodes in the lower paraaortic region.

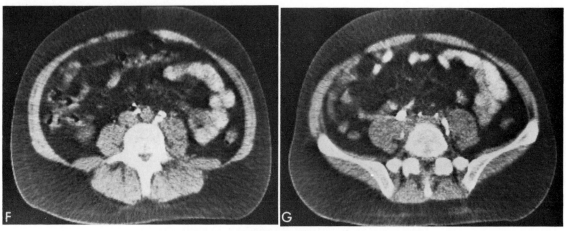

FIGURE 5–2f, g

Normal nodes are distributed around the aorta and the inferior vena cava. No enlargement of mesenteric nodes is demonstrated. What about these three sections of the pelvis?

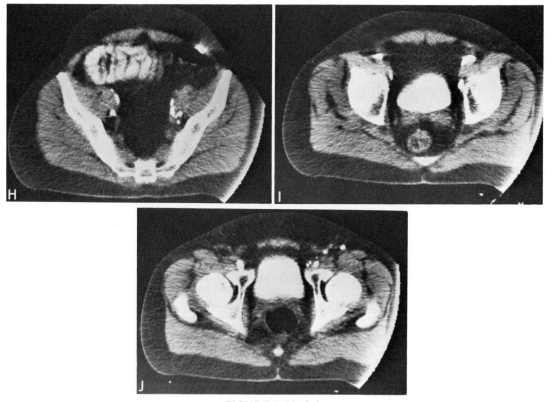

FIGURE 5–2h, i, j

The opacified nodes lie near the iliac vessels and the medial aspects of the iliopsoas muscles on section *h*. More inferiorly the opacified nodes lie near the external iliac vessels. Still more distally the opacified nodes are superficial in position along with the femoral vessels. The deep pelvic nodes are not generally opacified by pedal lymphography but can be seen by CT scan when they are enlarged.

The CT scan and the lymphogram often have a role in the evaluation of the lymph nodes. The lymphogram details only certain node groups, depending on the injection site and individual variations in anatomy. However, it does demonstrate the internal architecture of the nodes that are opacified so that subtle abnormalities can be detected before there is nodal enlargement or gross deformity. Occasionally the nature of the internal nodal derangement will be rather specific for a certain disease process.

The CT scan, on the other hand, depends exclusively on nodal enlargement to determine abnormality and is completely nonspecific. Occasionally, following lymphography, gross distortion of a node without accompanying enlargement is seen at CT scanning.

The primary uses of CT in the evaluation of lymph nodes are to study nodes in areas not normally opacified by lymphography, such as the celiac nodes, the splenic, mesenteric and hepatic nodes and the retrocrural nodes and to better demonstrate the extent of adenopathy found during lymphography. When massive adenopathy is suspected clinically, CT can be used to confirm this impression, and lymphography can be bypassed in certain patients.

CASE 5–3:

MR. C. G.

Mr. C. G. is a middle aged musician with a recent diagnosis of lymphoma made by supraclavicular node biopsy. You think he probably has widespread disease and are staging his disease prior to deciding on the appropriate therapy. You decide to do a CT scan because a lymphogram would not be necessary, if there is massive adenopathy. Several sections from this study are illustrated. What observations can you make?

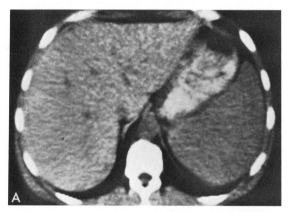

FIGURE 5–3a

This section shows massive splenomegaly, and you should also wonder about hepatic enlargement. No intrinsic abnormalities are seen in either liver or spleen and no enlarged retrocrural nodes are present.

The next section is from an area about 6 cm distal to the first. Now what do you see?

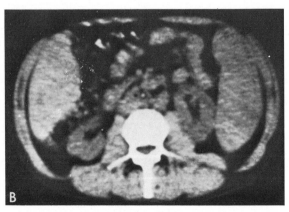

FIGURE 5–3b

The enlarged spleen is still seen and is actually compressing the left kidney, obscuring the fat planes between the kidney and the spleen and the kidney and the left psoas muscle. The paraaortic nodes are moderately enlarged but there is no massive adenopathy.

The remainder of the examination shows some enlarged nodes. It is decided that Mr. C. G. should have a lymphogram, since the presence of multiple rather discrete enlarged nodes at CT scanning could be caused by fatty replacement or other inflammatory change. Before the lymphogram is done you complete the splenic and the hepatic CT evaluations with scans done after contrast medium infusion. What do you see on this section?

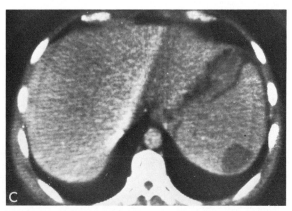

FIGURE 5-3c

There is a low attenuation, wedge-shaped defect in the spleen. An artifact crosses the liver but it is otherwise normal. The peripheral splenic defect may be a lymphomatous deposit but can also be caused by a splenic infarct.

A pedal lymphogram on Mr. C. G. shows many abnormal nodes 1 to 2 cm in size. A limited CT scan is performed after the lymphogram to correlate the findings. Two sections are illustrated. What do you see?

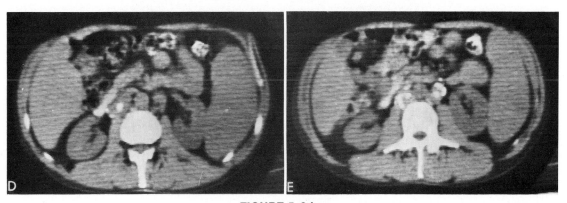

FIGURE 5-3d, e

The CT technique has been changed and these scans are easier to evaluate than the initial studies. Some oral contrast medium has also been given for this examination. The lymphographic contrast medium is seen in the paraaortic nodes, which were called abnormal on the earlier study.

A very important observation is the irregular or selective nodal filling that is achieved. Only a portion of the enlarged nodes present are demonstrated by lymphography. This fact means that in selected patients CT scanning can aid in radiation therapy port planning because it defines the extent of adenopathy more precisely than does lymphography.

CASE 5–4:

MR. F. G.

Mr. F. G. is a 77 year old patient of yours who does not come in for regular checkups. When he turns up after several years, he is limping and his right leg is very swollen. He also mentions that he hasn't been feeling well. You examine him with increasing apprehension because, in addition to his swollen right leg, he has a hard right inguinal mass, hepatosplenomegaly, possible abdominal masses and cervical adenopathy. You have a cervical node biopsy performed that reveals lymphocytic lymphoma. Mr F. G.'s disease is obviously widespread, so you order an abdominal CT scan to check the extent of disease. Selected sections are illustrated. What do you see on the first one?

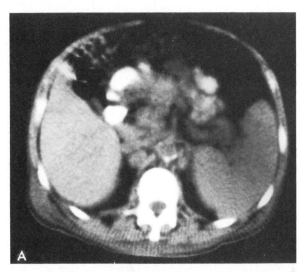

FIGURE 5–4a

The spleen is enlarged but shows no filling defects. There are poorly defined lobular densities in the splenic hilum that may be enlarged lymph nodes, but differentiation of nodes from splenic veins is always difficult. Enlarged nodes are present around the origin of the superior mesenteric artery. Complete evaluation of the liver does not show filling defects or an infiltrating lesion, but hepatomegaly is present. Serial scans reveal extensive mesenteric and retroperitoneal bulky adenopathy. The next scan illustrated is from the level of the renal pelves. What do you see?

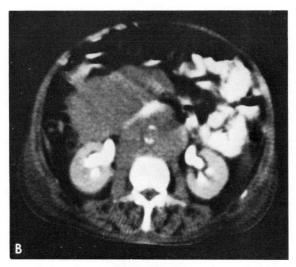

FIGURE 5–4b

The abnormalities are so extensive that it is hard to know where to begin. There is a large mesenteric mass and a second large retroperitoneal mass. The two are separated by contrast medium in the duodenum. Notice that the calcified aorta has been moved away from the spine by the extensive tumor. This is not a specific sign for tumor, since a leaking aortic aneurysm or any other cause of increased retroperitoneal tissue can cause the aorta to move anteriorly. Both renal pelves are quite full and have been rotated anteriorly by the massive adenopathy. You continue the study, and the next illustrated scan is just below the aortic bifurcation. What do you see here?

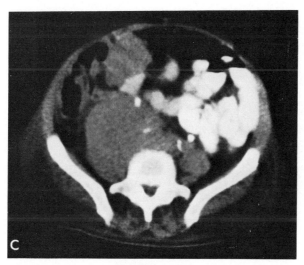

FIGURE 5–4c

The retroperitoneal disease has become quite asymmetrical and you speculate that the tumor mass on the right is causing Mr. F. G.'s right leg edema. The right ureter is displaced very far anterior while the left is in nearly normal position. The intraperitoneal mass is quite small at this level. The next scan is in the true pelvis. What do you see now?

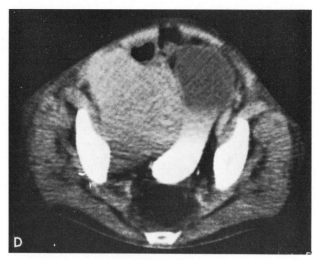

FIGURE 5–4d

The urinary bladder is markedly displaced to the left by a large right sided soft tissue mass. No nodal abnormality is seen on the left at this level. Mr. F. G.'s bladder is so large that you wonder about outlet obstruction. He says he has had a diminution of urinary stream and increased nocturnal frequency. The next section is just above the symphysis pubis. What are the findings here?

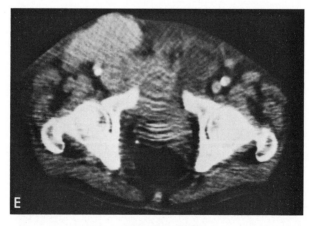

FIGURE 5–4e

The right-sided abnormality persists as the prominent inguinal mass that you felt. Calcification in the femoral artery lets you know that the neurovascular bundle is surrounded by tumor, undoubtedly contributing to the leg edema. There is a circular computer artifact obscuring the prostate, which is also enlarged. What about the final section?

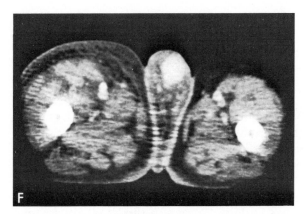

FIGURE 5–4f

This section in mid-thigh illustrates the diffuse swelling of the right leg. Individual muscle bellies are clearly larger on the right than on the left. Again computer artifact obscures subtle detail. This type of artifact is seen primarily with scanners that have a circular array of detectors.

Mr. F. G. responds well to initial chemotherapy and decides to take a cruise around the world. You do not see him again.

CASE 5–5:

MR. W. K.

Mr. W. K., a cantankerous millionaire on the board of your hospital, demands to be seen at once. Usually his complaints are more imagined than real, but today he complains of weight loss, fever, cramping, abdominal pain and diarrhea. After drawing routine blood counts and serum chemistries, you perform a physical examination. There is splenomegaly and diffuse abdominal fullness. You order an upper gastrointestinal series and barium enema and are startled when you review the examinations. What do you make of the illustrated films?

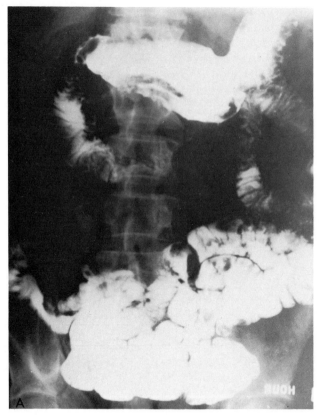

FIGURE 5–5a

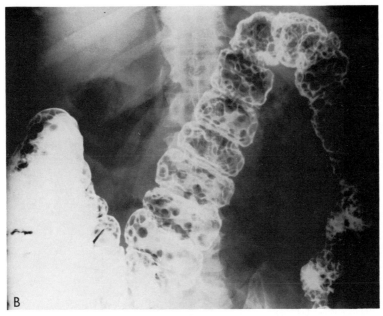

FIGURE 5–5b

There are diffusely thickened folds in the stomach and many poly-poid filling defects in the small bowel. The colon is carpeted with in-numerable sessile polyps. A biopsy reveals lymphoma and you order a CT scan to evaluate the extent of disease. What information is obtained in this first section at the level of the xyphoid? Both oral and intravenous contrast media have been given.

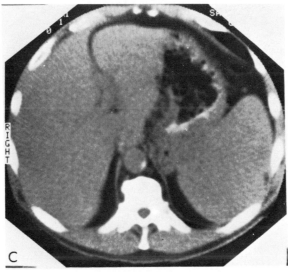

FIGURE 5–5c

The liver is normal in size and consistency. The gastric wall seems thickened, but this is a difficult observation to evaluate when the stomach is not completely distended. Most of the contrast medium is in the gastric antrum seen on scan *d* and the fundus is only partially distended by gas. The spleen is enlarged and displaces the stomach medially. What is seen on the next section?

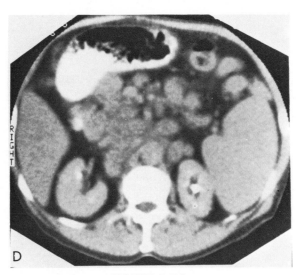

FIGURE 5–5d

The gastric antrum and a small portion of the duodenum are opacified by contrast medium. Between the stomach and the aorta and inferior vena cava there is a large group of ovoid soft tissue densities. These are enlarged and somewhat matted retroperitoneal and mesenteric lymph nodes. The enlarged but homogeneous spleen is pressing upon the lateral aspect of the left kidney. The next section is more caudal. Is it abnormal?

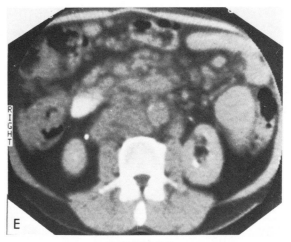

FIGURE 5–5e

Again there is extensive retroperitoneal and mesenteric adenopathy. While the aorta can be seen, the inferior vena cava is obscured by the enlarged, matted nodes and the right ureter is displaced laterally. The inferior aspect of the spleen lies between the left kidney and the gas-containing descending colon. What additional abnormality is seen on the next section?

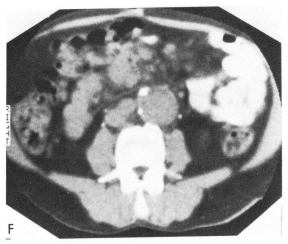

FIGURE 5–5f

Both mesenteric and retroperitoneal adenopathy are still demonstrated. An aneurysm of the abdominal aorta is seen at this level.

Clearly, Mr. W. K. has a very extensive lymphoma but his response to chemotherapy is dramatic. He departs for his summer home in Bora-Bora, where he dies 18 months later. So impressed was he with the CT scanner that he left part of his fortune for further modernization of the radiology department.

CASE 5–6:

MR. N. B.

Episodic gross total hematuria and left flank pain bring Mr. N. B., a 52 year old man, to see you. Intravenous urogram demonstrates an abnormal left kidney. It has function but is markedly enlarged, and the collecting system is distorted. The left ureter is displaced anteriorly on the oblique films. This finding is quite disturbing and so you order a CT scan to evaluate the retroperitoneum. Three sections done after both intravenous and oral contrast media have been given are demonstrated. What do you see on the first scan?

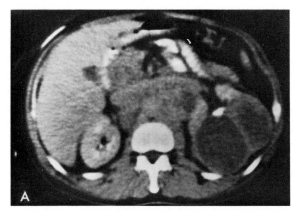

FIGURE 5–6a

The left kidney is enlarged and has two areas of low attenuation. The more dorsal one has a sharp margin and you think this is probably a renal cyst. The second, more ventral, area of low attenuation has a thick, irregular shaggy wall. These findings suggest a necrotic renal cell carcinoma. The kidney has rotated so that the renal pelvis is on the ventral surface. The aorta and the inferior vena cava are completely obscured by a soft tissue mass. What do you see on the next two scans?

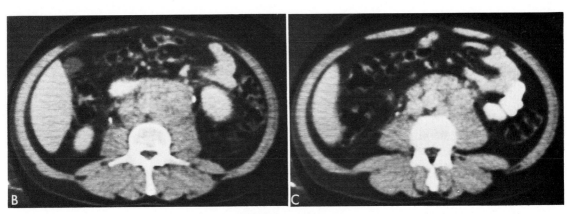

FIGURE 5–6b, c

The bulky retroperitoneal adenopathy is present on both sections. The opacified left ureter is displaced both ventrally and laterally by the nodal mass. Though massive retroperitoneal adenopathy is present on section *c*, the aorta and the inferior vena cava can be distinguished.

A left radical nephrectomy is performed because of the persistent hematuria. The renal cell carcinoma and the renal cyst are confirmed. During the operation an attempt is made to resect all the involved nodes. Information proved by the CT scan influenced the decision to use an anterior approach and aided in planning the extent of the nodal exploration.

CASE 5-7:

MRS. D. S.

Mrs. D. S., a middle aged woman who is active in several civic projects, has been feeling "run down" for several months. She has found masses in both groins and thinks that there are also some in her axillae. A biopsy reveals an undifferentiated lymphoma. She is referred to you for therapy. In addition to the axillary and inguinal adenopathy, you find dullness in both lung bases and a vague fullness in the mid-abdomen. Since she clearly has extensive disease, you order a CT scan to evaluate the paraaortic and pelvic lymph nodes. The examination is performed after oral and intravenous contrast material have been administered. Representative sections are illustrated. What are your conclusions?

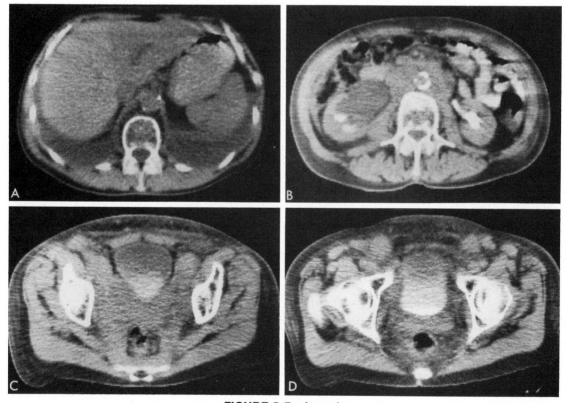

FIGURE 5-7a, b, c, d

As you suspected, Mrs. D. S. has extensive abdominal and pelvic lymphadenopathy. The bladder is actually compressed. The palpable adenopathy in the inguinal regions is well seen. There are two additional observations you should have made. The first of these is a finding not previously encountered in these exercises. The dullness you found in both lung bases is explained by large bilateral pleural effusions. These cause the crescentic homogeneous areas of increased attenuation in the posterior costophrenic sulci on section a. The second observation is the right-sided hydronephrosis seen on section b.

After much discussion with the patient and her family and considerable consultation with colleagues, it is decided to try the patient on cyclic chemotherapy with a reevaluation of the patient both by clinical examination and by a repeat CT scan after the initial course of therapy.

Two weeks later, you see the patient after the first course of treatment. She feels better and the CT scan has been repeated. The new sections illustrated should be compared to the sections at similar levels. Is there objective evidence of response to treatment?

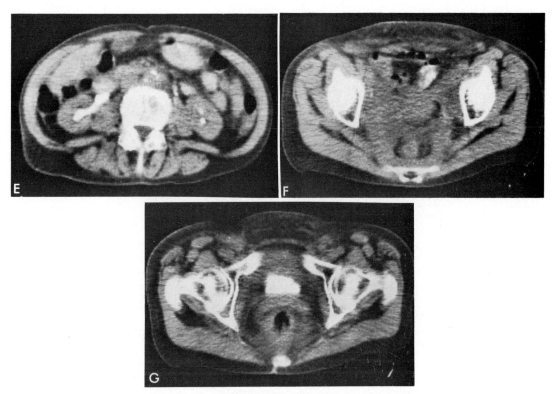

FIGURE 5–7e, f, g

While there is persistent abnormality at every level, the bulk of the adenopathy is clearly diminished. The right hydronephrosis has completely resolved. It is decided to continue therapy with careful clinical supervision.

This case illustrates the facility with which CT can evaluate the extent of adenopathy, a point that has been emphasized previously. It is an ideal modality for the sequential evaluation of the efficacy of a particular therapeutic method. In this setting, the CT examination can be confined to the areas of greatest abnormality and can be quite brief.

CASE 5–8:

MRS. K. T.

Mrs. K. T. is a 39 year old woman who became your patient about 18 months ago. At that time she saw her internist for back pain and spine films showed a destructive lesion of the right side of the L4 vertebral body. Biopsy of the vertebra led to a diagnosis of leiomyosarcoma. No primary lesion was found, but radiation therapy was given in an attempt to decrease her back pain. You have been following her ever since.

The radiation therapy did decrease her back pain for some months, though she has never been really free of pain. Recently her discomfort has been increasing and she is using large amounts of pain medication. You decide it is time to reevaluate the tumor, so you request a CT scan of the retroperitoneum. The first scan is at the level of L4. No contrast material has been given. What do you see?

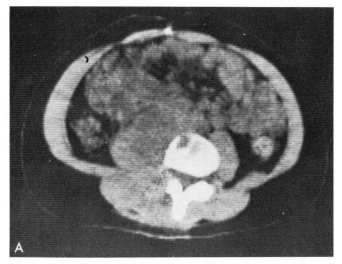

FIGURE 5–8a

The destructive lesion of L4 is seen, though the mean and window are set for the optimum soft tissue demonstration. A bone setting shows much greater destruction than is apparent here. You have been observing the bone lesion by x-ray and are more concerned about the new bulky soft tissue mass anterior and lateral to the spine. The mass has engulfed and enlarged the right psoas muscle and is obscuring the iliac arteries and veins.

The mass extends distally for several centimeters but does not extend cranially very far. You wonder what the mass has done to the right ureter, so you do a scan at the level of the kidneys. Oral contrast medium has been given to help evaluate the true extent of the mass, but intravenous contrast medium has not been given because of a history of a previous severe reaction to contrast material. What do you see?

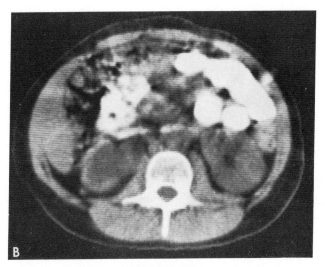

FIGURE 5–8b

The left kidney is normal, but the right one has parenchymal thinning and dilatation of the collecting system. The right renal pelvis is partly extrarenal and is quite dilated. The degree of parenchymal loss indicates that the obstruction is long standing. The psoas muscles are normal at this level. There is a soft tissue nodule dorsal to the right kidney that could be a tumor nodule or a dilated collateral vein. Palliative therapy is about all that can be offered Mrs. K. T. and so you do not pursue investigation of this nodule.

CASE 5–9:

MR. T. K.

Your patient Mr. T. K. is again referred to you because of increasing abdominal girth. One year ago he underwent operation in an attempt to remove a large retroperitoneal liposarcoma. The tumor could not be completely resected and following surgery he had a course of radiotherapy. Now he has abdominal pain and he can no longer buckle his belt. On physical examination he has several large masses in his abdomen. It is clear that Mr. T. K. has recurrent tumor, so you order an abdominal CT scan to assess its extent.

The initial scan illustrated was done after oral and intravenous contrast media were given. What areas are abnormal?

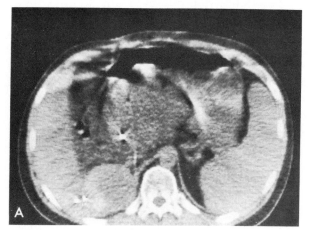

FIGURE 5–9a

The body and antrum of the stomach are draped over a rather large mass with multiple lobulations in the region of the body and head of the pancreas. Several metallic clips have caused spray artifacts, as has the gas in the transverse colon. There is dilute contrast material in the duodenum adjacent to the mass. A round mass is intimately applied to the medial surface of the liver posteriorly and also to the right crus of the diaphragm, which is thickened. The spleen is enlarged, probably because of venous obstruction. The next section is more caudal. What information is added?

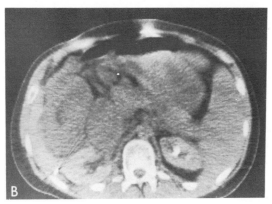

FIGURE 5–9b

A surgical clip is seen lateral to the right kidney, which is compressed by two large masses on its anterior surface. In the mid and left abdomen there is a large ovoid mass that extends toward the anterior abdominal wall. Three more scans are shown. What is the extent of the intraabdominal mass?

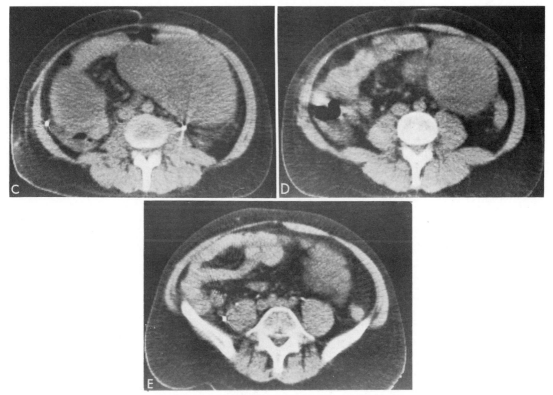

FIGURE 5–9c, d, e

It is clear that the larger mass extends down below the level of the iliac crest. The smaller one ends in mid-abdomen. On the basis of the diagnosis of intraabdominal and retroperitoneal recurrence, it is decided to reexplore Mr. T. K. to remove as much tumor as possible. He realizes that a cure is not possible but thinks surgery will make his life more comfortable at the moment.

CT scanning provides a simple way to fully determine the extent of such soft tissue lesions. While ultrasound will suffice in some patients, such massive disease is often best evaluated by CT.

CASE 5–10:

MR. M. S.

Mr. M. S. is a fragile 73 year old man who has claudication in his left leg. He has no peripheral pulses on the left and none below the common femoral artery on the right; also, you feel a pulsatile abdominal mass. Since an abdominal aortic aneurysm would influence both your diagnostic and surgical approach, you order an ultrasound of the abdominal aorta. Ultrasound generally gives a very good demonstration of the abdominal aorta and will demonstrate clotted aneurysms better than angiography. However, because Mr. M. S. has extensive bowel gas, a satisfactory study cannot be obtained. You still hope to avoid angiography in this frail man so you order a CT scan, which is done prior to and following the infusion of intravenous contrast medium. One scan done before the contrast material infusion and two after are illustrated. What do you see?

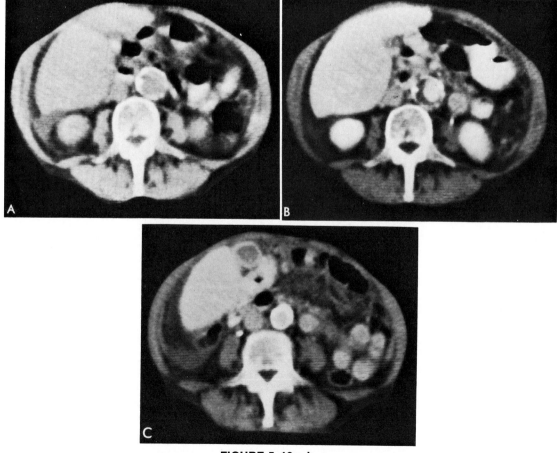

FIGURE 5–10a, b, c

The noncontrast medium scan *a* shows a small amount of ascites beside the liver, an unexpected finding. The abdominal aorta is heavily calcified and measures about 3.5 cm in transverse diameter. Slight artifacts are caused by peristalsis. Scan *b* shows the contrast medium in the aortic lumen surrounded by a low attenuation halo. This is a mural thrombus. The second scan done near the aortic bifurcation shows very heavy wall calcification but no further thrombus. The thrombus extends from just below the renal arteries for about 5 cm. Incidentally, did you notice the thick gallbladder wall on *c*? Mr. M. S. has had fatty food intolerance for years.

Mr. M. S. feels well at bed rest in the hospital so he refuses surgery and signs out. A few months later you see his sister and she reports that Mr. M. S. has died. Apparently, the ascites seen on the CT scan was the first evidence of carcinomatosis from a colonic primary lesion.

MR. R. F.

Mr. R. F. is a 65 year old man with severe atherosclerotic vascular disease who had resection of an abdominal aortic aneurysm five years ago. Angiography at that time demonstrated elongated iliac arteries. He has been reasonably well but now is being evaluated for a transurethral prostatectomy. An intravenous urogram has been ordered to demonstrate the upper collecting systems. The preliminary film is illustrated. What do you see?

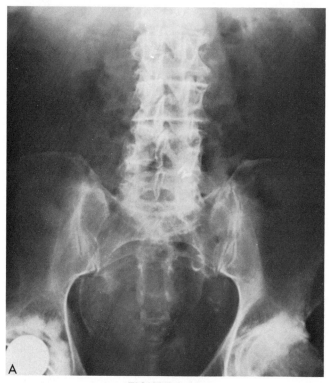

FIGURE 5–11a

Mr. R. F. seems to be wearing out. He has severe degenerative disease of his lumbar spine and left hip. He already has had a right hip replacement. Surgical clips from his aortic aneurysm resection are overlying L5. More important is a rounded calcified mass primarily in the right hemipelvis. What might this be? How do you plan to approach its diagnosis?

First, you review the remainder of the intravenous urogram, which shows only displacement of the right ureter. Next you order a pelvic ultrasound. This demonstrates the mass well and shows some internal echoes suggesting that the mass might be solid. However, the calcification in the wall of the mass causes shadowing, so the ultrasonographer will not give you a dogmatic statement about the mass. A barium enema shows only extrinsic impression, as does a small bowel series. To sum up your evidence, you are dealing with a mass with wall calcification that has arisen in five years. It is extrinsic to the colon and the genitourinary tract. It seems solid on ultrasound. You finally order a CT scan to try to delineate the mass better. What do you see on the first section?

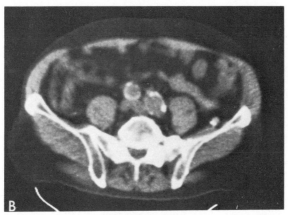

FIGURE 5–11b

The scan shows calcification in both common iliac arteries. Both are dilated, but the left is larger than the right. The second section is about 6 cm lower. What observations can you make?

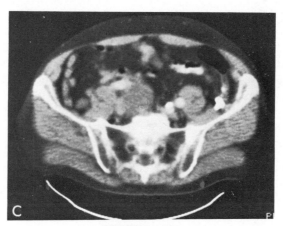

FIGURE 5–11c

The mass is now seen on the right. It does appear to be solid by CT criteria. The contrast medium-filled left internal and external iliac arteries are seen with a coarse calcification between them. On the right only a single channel is opacified and it is ventral and lateral to the mass. Does the third section add any information?

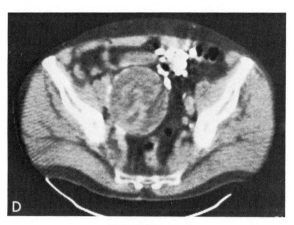

FIGURE 5–11d

The mass seems somewhat mottled on this section and the calcific rim is well seen. The external iliac arteries are difficult to identify but appear to be separate from the mass. What are your conclusions?

The appearance over a five year interval of a mass with curvilinear rim calcification in a man with severe vascular disease should make you strongly suspect an aneurysm from the start of your investigation. The solid appearance at ultrasound and then at CT scanning should suggest clot in an aneurysm. The mottled appearance on the final section illustrated implies that there is still a patent channel through the aneurysm. At this point, however, you really cannot give a dogmatic diagnosis, since some connective tissue tumors can have peripheral calcification of this nature. Though you feel aneurysm is the most likely diagnosis, arteriography is performed.

Transaxillary aortography demonstrates a very irregular channel in a large right internal iliac artery aneurysm nearly filled with clot.

CT SCANNING
IN THE ABDOMEN

The barium examination is the primary radiographic modality for the hollow viscera of the abdomen. Mucosal and mural lesions of these organs are well seen with this technique and CT has little to offer. Mass lesions that arise in the hollow viscera but grow extrinsically can be detected by conventional techniques, but the full extent of such masses can be difficult to determine. CT scanning can add useful information in these patients. CT is also of value in demonstrating lesions that arise in the mesentery or in nongastrointestinal abdominal organs and invade or displace the bowel.

The area of the abdomen to be examined will be determined by the earlier examinations. The adjacent or involved small bowel should be opacified with dilute contrast material. Because it is important not to confuse normal gastrointestinal contents with pathologic masses, it may be necessary to withhold food before the examination. In a large hollow viscus such as the stomach, the decubitus view may be helpful in separating gastric contents from a true mass. Decubitus views are also useful in demonstrating the normal mobility of bowel loops or a viscus.

CT scanning specifically for the contents of the abdominal cavity is an ancillary procedure that should be performed only when it is felt that useful information may be obtained. However, whenever the abdomen or the retroperitoneum is examined by CT, the abdominal contents are included and should be evaluated.

Since the abdominal contents have been repeatedly illustrated in the cases presented earlier in this book, no specific normal abdomen illustrations are presented. A few examples of intraabdominal pathology demonstrated by CT scanning are illustrated. It cannot be stressed enough that at present CT has a very limited role in the evaluation of hollow viscera, mesentery and omentum. When a CT examination is performed for these organs, it must be designed for the situation at hand.

CASE 6–1:

MR. B. H.

Mr. B. H. is a 40 year old man who sees you because of increasing abdominal girth. Physical examination demonstrates ascites and a diagnostic paracentesis yields malignant cells. Routine examinations do not reveal the primary malignancy, so a CT scan is ordered to attempt to find a mass. Although the CT scan does not answer this question, Mr. B. H.'s scan is a good example of the CT appearance of extensive ascites. Three scans are illustrated.

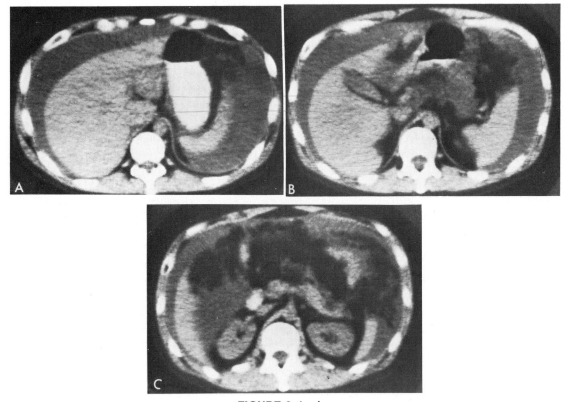

FIGURE 6–1a, b, c

Ascites surrounds the liver laterally, displacing it medially. The spleen is also displaced medially, and on scans *b* and *c*, the bowel is seen floating centrally in the ascitic fluid. The retroperitoneal fat planes and the pancreatic tail are well seen. The right adrenal gland is seen on section *a* and the left on *b*.

Ascites can be generalized as in this patient or may localize, as in Case 5–9, in one or several areas for no apparent reason.

Mr. B. H. is discharged on palliative chemotherapy without a diagnosis. A few months later increasing loss of appetite prompts a repeat upper gastrointestinal series. Changes of linitis plastica are present; this observation is confirmed by biopsy.

Miss A. F. comes to your office complaining of left abdominal pain. She is an obese middle aged woman who has recently taken up bike riding to try to lose weight, but the exercise only improves her appetite. She had a rather bad spill two days ago, hitting her left side on a curb. On physical examination the area is tender and a vague fullness is present in the left abdomen. Her blood profile shows a drop in hemoglobin from previous examinations. You are concerned about splenic injury and so you order an ultrasound for splenic rupture. The patient's body habitus and bowel gas greatly limit the study; a CT scan is suggested as an alternative. Two scans are illustrated. What is the abnormality?

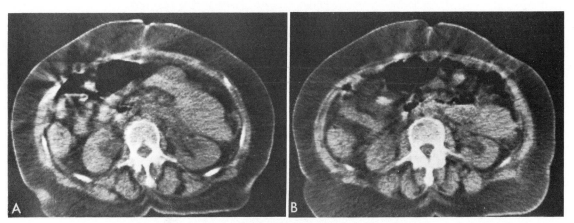

FIGURE 6–2a, b

There is a large fusiform area of increased attenuation in the left abdomen anterior to the left kidney but definitely separate from it. The mass extends to the midline and is adjacent to bowel. Its location and shape suggest that it is confined by the mesentery. The CT number is high enough to exclude a lipoma or serous fluid collection. Scans of the spleen are normal, as was the remainder of the abdomen.

Since Miss A. F. continues to have pain, surgery is decided upon. A large intramesenteric hematoma is evacuated and Miss A. F. has a normal convalescence. She decides to forego bicycling. When you next see her, she has regained the weight she lost during her stay in the hospital.

MR. S. N.

Mr. S. N. has had a spiking fever for four days and you are sure he has an intraabdominal abscess. Two weeks ago he had a partial gastrectomy and splenectomy for a perforated giant gastric ulcer. The initial postoperative course was quite smooth and the drains were removed after eight days. Now, because there are diminished breath sounds at the left lung base, you obtain a chest film. What do you see?

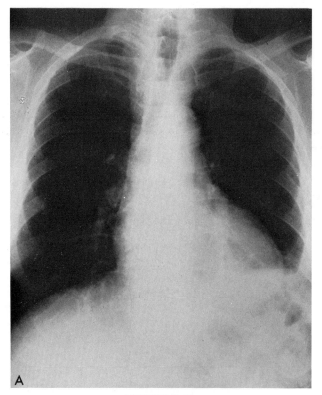

FIGURE 6–3a

A left pleural effusion and some streaky atelectasis behind the heart are noted. The left hemidiaphragm is not elevated. More important, there are several amorphous gas collections beneath the left hemidiaphragm. The remainder of the chest film is unchanged from earlier examinations. The radiologist fluoroscopes the diaphragm and reports diminished excursions on the left. A left subphrenic abscess, which could have occurred after his operation, could be causing Mr. S. N.'s signs and symptoms.

The gas in the left upper quadrant will interfere with an ultrasound so you order a CT scan to look for an abscess. Three sections from the CT scan are illustrated. What do you see on the first section? Oral and intravenous contrast material have both been given.

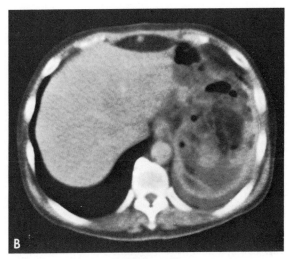

FIGURE 6–3b

This section is somewhat difficult to interpret by itself, but you should make several observations. The left pleural effusion is seen dorsal to the diaphragm. The diaphragm itself is thickened. Anterior to the diaphragm is an extensive amorphous collection. Several gas pockets are present and there are air fluid levels. None of this soft tissue can be clearly identified as bowel. You should suspect that most, if not all, of this collection is an abscess, but you must look at additional sections before reaching a definite conclusion. What do you see on the next scan?

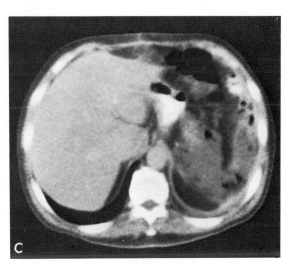

FIGURE 6–3c

Two irregularly shaped collections, which contain gas and fluid, are present in the left abdomen. Dilated bowel loops are seen ventral to these collections and there is contrast medium in the small gastric remnant. The left hemidiaphragm again appears thickened. You can compare it to the normal one on the right. What abnormality is on the final section?

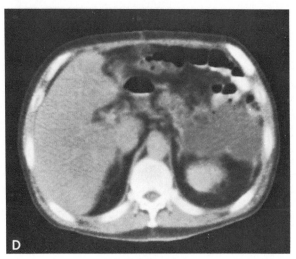

FIGURE 6–3d

At this level the top of the left kidney is seen. Ventral to it is an irregular, nonhomogeneous soft tissue collection containing fluid and some gas. Dilated bowel loops are again seen. The radiologist tells you he thinks the patient has a large amorphous abscess that seems to have a horseshoe configuration. It extends from the level of the left kidney to the diaphragm, occupying much of the left upper quadrant. You take Mr. S. N. back to surgery and drain a large multilocular abscess located in the splenic bed and lesser sac areas. He has an uneventful but lengthy convalescence.

The extent of the abscess is very well defined with CT scanning. In some patients ultrasound will do as well, but when gas and other bowel contents are present, CT scanning is the better technique.

Mr. A. G. is a 65 year old man who comes in for a routine physical examination. He has no complaints and looks very healthy. You are surprised to palpate a firm, round left upper quadrant mass. Laboratory tests do not help in your diagnosis, so you order an intravenous urogram. What do you see?

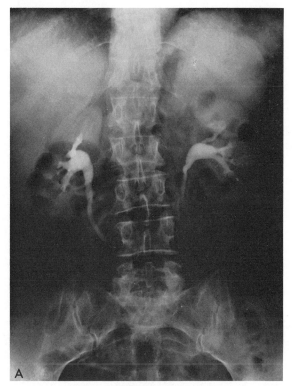

FIGURE 6–4a

The renal contours and collecting systems are normal but there is a rounded mass measuring about 10 cm in diameter in the left upper quadrant. The mass does not appear to arise from the left kidney, so you order a barium enema and upper gastrointestinal series. The barium enema shows only an extrinsic impression on the transverse colon. What do you see on this film from the gastrointestinal series?

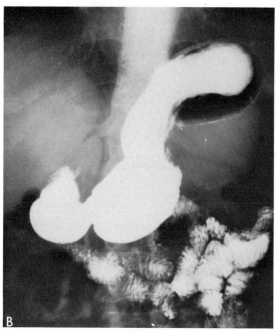

FIGURE 6–4b

The mass is impressing on the greater curvature but does not disturb the gastric mucosal pattern. Some jejunum is displaced inferiorly.

You still have no idea about the nature of the mass or which organ it arises from. Certainly, it must be operated upon but the surgeon would like to know more about what he is getting into, so you suggest a CT scan to see if you can answer any of his questions. Two scans are illustrated. What, if any, conclusions can you reach?

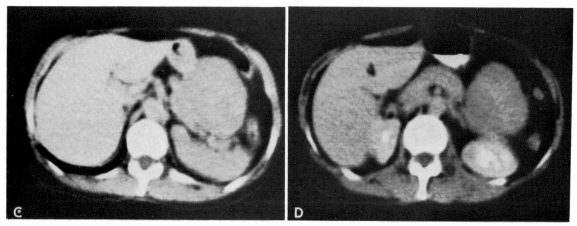

FIGURE 6–4c, d

The mass is seen on both sections and is quite homogeneous. On section c you can see that it is separate from the spleen. It also does not arise from the kidney. On section d the pancreas can be separated from the mass, but it does compress the pancreatic tail. The mass is inseparable from the stomach and could conceivably arise from the wall of the stomach.

The surgeon is resigned to operating on the mass without a more definite diagnosis. Both you and he are pleased when he finds a pedunculated gastric leiomyoma. Mr. A. G. is overjoyed to learn he does not have cancer and goes to Acapulco to convalesce.

While it is reasonable to try to determine the organ of origin of a mass, this is often difficult at CT when a large mass adjacent to many structures compresses the fat planes that normally demarcate the various organs.

CASE 6–5:

MRS. G. R.

Mrs. G. R. is a 62 year old woman who had a right colectomy 18 months ago for a large cecal carcinoma. She has been feeling well, but four or five weeks ago she began to have a full feeling in her abdomen along with some rather vague abdominal distress. Physical examination is not very helpful but does suggest fullness of her lower abdomen compared to earlier examinations. Since several lymph nodes were positive in the surgical specimen, you expect tumor recurrence, but upper gastrointestinal series with small bowel follow-through, barium enema and intravenous urogram have all been rather unhelpful. The most disturbing small bowel film is shown. Do you see any abnormality?

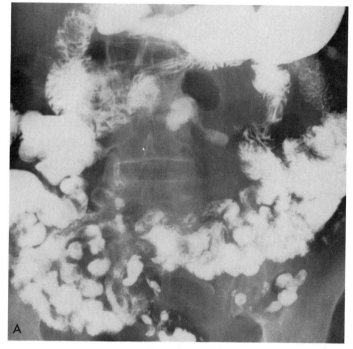

FIGURE 6–5a

The small bowel seems to be displaced from the mid-abdomen but a definite mass is not seen.

Still concerned about tumor recurrence, you order a CT scan of the abdomen. Oral and intravenous contrast media have been given. The upper abdomen is normal but sections below the umbilicus are not. What do you see on this section 6 cm below the umbilicus?

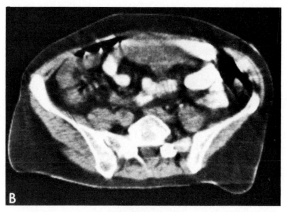

FIGURE 6–5b

The first thing that should catch your attention is a lobulated soft tissue mass adherent to the anterior abdominal wall. Small bowel filled with contrast material is adjacent to the tumor mass but does not seem to be entrapped by it. In addition, there is another rounded mass medial to the right psoas muscle, caused by tumor in prevertebral lymph nodes.

The tumor recurrence is confirmed by fine needle transabdominal biopsy and Mrs. G. R. is placed on chemotherapy.

CASE 6–6:

MISS P. O.

Miss P. O., an unfortunate 32 year old woman with metastatic melanoma, is about to be placed on an experimental chemotherapy protocol. Prior to this you need to know the true extent of her disease. She has widespread pulmonary metastases. You plan to do a series of abdominal examinations but Miss P. O. is understandably reluctant to undergo more tests. For this reason, you order an abdominal CT scan. Intravenous and oral contrast material have been given. The first section was taken through the upper abdomen. What do you see?

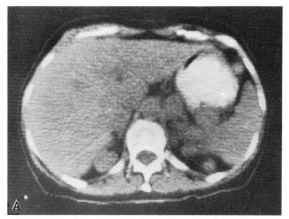

FIGURE 6–6a

The liver and the spleen are normal but there are two nodules on the serosal surface of the stomach. There are multiple rounded masses in the retroperitoneal fat adjacent to the aorta and dorsal to the spleen.

What abnormalities do you see in this next section?

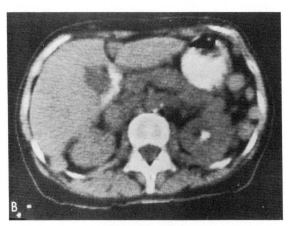

FIGURE 6–6b

There are many more nodules. Those in the fat lateral to the stomach and left kidney are particularly obvious. Also, a large nodule is present posterior to the right lobe of the liver; another nodule is seen in the cleft between the right and left lobes. A small subcutaneous nodule and several paraaortic nodules are also demonstrated.

The next two sections are taken through the lower abdomen and the upper pelvis. Again the abnormalities are dramatic.

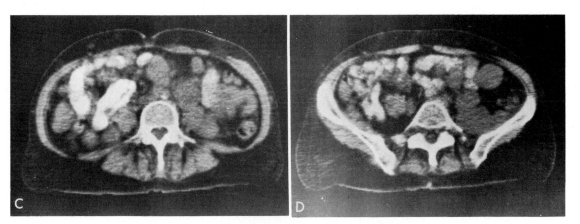

FIGURE 6–6c, d

Innumerable nodules involve the paraaortic region, the retroperitoneum, the mesenteric fat and serosal surface of the bowel. The final section is from a location in the mid-pelvis.

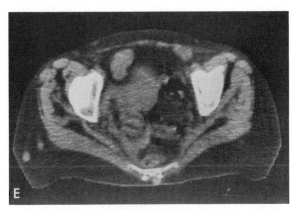

FIGURE 6–6e

There are two nodules in the fat of the right buttock and two prominent nodules in the peritoneal fat just behind the rectus sheath. Inguinal adenopathy is present on the right. The section includes the tip of the uterine fundus.

You are surprised by the extent of occult metastatic disease. In spite of this large tumor burden, Miss P. O. seems to respond well to chemotherapy.

It is apparent that CT is very successful in the demonstration of this kind of soft tissue abnormality. Indeed, there is no other technique that can provide this type of information.

CT SCANNING
OF THE PELVIS

The primary diagnostic modality for evaluation of the pelvis is ultra-sound. It can differentiate solid from cystic masses with great accuracy. Since it does not employ ionizing radiation, it is very useful in the evaluation of problem pregnancies and in the reproductive age group in general. Pelvic ultrasound depends on full distention of the urinary bladder, which acts as a window for sound transmission and displaces bowel from the pelvis. When the bladder cannot be distended, the study will be limited at best and is often not possible. The pelvic side walls are also not well examined with ultrasound. CT becomes a useful technique in evaluation of the pelvis in patients with masses involving the pelvic side wall, with pelvic bony abnormalities and when the bladder cannot be distended. In the reproductive age group, pelvic CT scanning must be used with care, since it does involve radiation.

It is in the evaluation of pelvic malignancy that CT has its major applications. The transaxial tomograms provide excellent definition of organ boundaries and tissue planes, permitting evaluation of spread of a neoplastic process beyond the organ of origin. The many pelvic lymph nodes, including those not seen at lymphography, can be examined for enlargement.

CT scanning may be used to study the nature and extent of a variety of pathologic processes involving the pelvic peritoneal cavity and the pelvic side walls. In certain situations, the sensitivity of CT to variations in tissue x-ray attenuation can provide specific information about fat or gas within a mass lesion.

Each CT scan of the pelvis must be tailored to the problem at hand. The number of scans, their position and frequency should be varied according to the questions that need to be answered. Use of organ markers or contrast media will also vary from patient to patient. When CT scanning of the pelvis is done appropriately it is a very useful diagnostic tool.

NORMAL PELVIC ANATOMY AND VARIATIONS

As in other areas of the body, the anatomy of the pelvis is quite variable from person to person. Anatomy of the reproductive organs varies with the sex and age of the patient.

The first sections are from an examination of a 40 year old woman. Look at both sections. What structures can you identify?

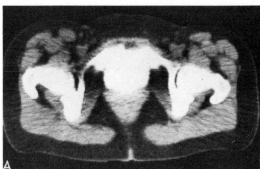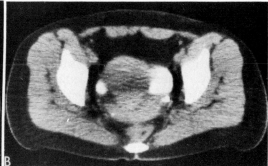

FIGURE 7–1a, b

Section *a* was made at the level of the femoral heads and pubic symphysis, through the pelvic floor. The bladder is opacified by contrast material. Behind the bladder is a triangular structure that is a composite of the vagina anteriorly and the distal rectum posteriorly. A tampon in the vagina will clearly identify it when needed. Lateral and posterior are the muscles and fat of the pelvic floor.

The second section shows a curious array of midline structures. The uterus is anteflexed and is lying against the dome of the bladder. Some of the opacified bladder is seen to each side of the uterus. There is a low attenuation artifact between the two parts of opacified bladder. The uterus not only varies in its basic orientation but its position changes with bladder distention. In this patient the uterus is being sectioned down its long axis; it resembles an inverted pear. The stem end is the lower uterine segment. The rectum is posterior and contains a small amount of gas. Between the uterus and the rectum are the laterally oriented adnexal structures. The high density structures next to the adnexa are phleboliths. It is not possible to distinguish the tubal and the ligamentous elements of the adnexa. The ovaries are occasionally seen.

The fat planes separating the midline structures from the muscular and bony pelvic side walls are of great diagnostic significance. Note the symmetrical appearance in this patient. The external iliac vessels and nodes are seen lying on the anterior aspect of the iliac bones. It is in this area that enlarged external iliac nodes would be sought. In the midline, ventrally, the paired rectus muscles are seen. Extraperitoneal fat separates these muscles from the bladder and uterus.

The next study was done after surgery on a 45 year old woman. What was the operation?

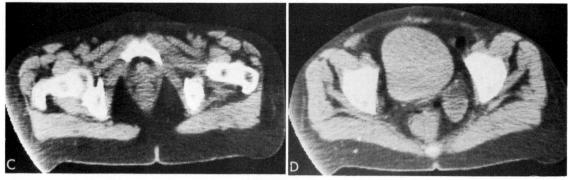

FIGURE 7-1c, d

Only the very tip of the bladder base is seen behind the symphysis. It has a slightly higher attenuation than the vagina and the distal rectum because of contrast medium. The vagina has a transverse orientation and the rectum is defined by fat.

The section through the mid-pelvis is more informative. The bladder is quite distended with opacified urine. Behind the bladder are the rectum and the sigmoid colon. The sigmoid colon extends anteriorly and to the left and contains some gas. The uterus and adnexa are not seen. The patient has had a hysterectomy and bilateral salpingo-oophorectomy.

The male pelvis has less fat, generally more muscle and a configuration that is somewhat different from the female pelvis. The sections illustrated are from an examination of a 26 year old man. What structures can you identify?

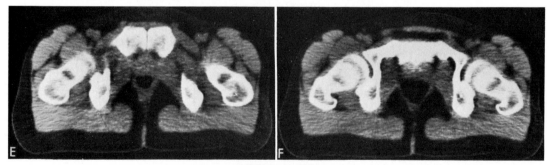

FIGURE 7-1e, f

Section *e* was made through the pubic symphysis. There is some fat separating the prostate gland from the symphysis anterior to it. The fat planes lateral to the prostate are not well defined on this section, and the gland seems to merge with the adjacent muscles. The rectum is posterior to the prostate. The anatomic plane of separation between the rectum and the prostate is not defined. Posterior and lateral to the rectum, there is a moderate amount of fat.

The next section is 1 cm cephalad to the first. Dense contrast material is in the base of the bladder. The prostate causes a bilobed impression on the bladder. The fat lateral to the prostate is well seen at this level, but the anterior rectal wall is inseparable from the prostatic capsule.

Section *g* is 2 cm higher. What new structures do you see?

Behind the bladder are the seminal vesicles. These have a bow tie-shaped configuration, extending out laterally between the bladder and the rectum. A fat plane separates the lateral lobes of the seminal vesicles from the posterior bladder wall. The dense contrast medium in the bladder obscures this fat plane on this section. The rectal ampulla is

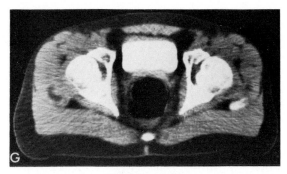

FIGURE 7-1g

distended by gas. There is a well defined fat plane that separates the bladder, the seminal vesicles and the rectum from the obturator internus muscles. These muscles form the pelvic side walls at this level.

The rectum and the sigmoid are generally present in the pelvis. The cecum, when low lying, may be seen in the right pelvis. The amount of bowel present in the pelvis depends in part on the distention of the bladder. This is well known in pelvic ultrasound, a technique which uses bladder distention to lift bowel out of the pelvis. Consider the next section. Oral contrast material has been given.

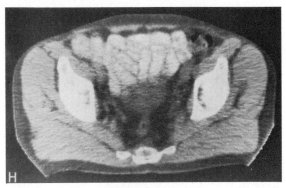

FIGURE 7-1h

There are many small bowel loops interposed between the bladder and the anterior abdominal wall. Ascites may also accumulate in this area. In very obese patients, abdominal contents may extend inferiorly over the pelvis. Look at the next section.

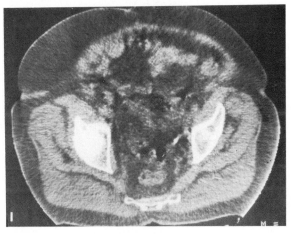

FIGURE 7-1i

Here, the very obese abdomen hangs down over the true pelvis. In this elderly man, only colon and rectum are seen on the section in addition to the small bowel.

CASE 7–2:

MR. N. R.

Mr. N. R. is an elderly, somewhat senile man who resides in a chronic care facility. His doctors think that he has developed a large pelvic mass so a CT scan is ordered. Three sections are illustrated. Intravenous contrast material has been given. What is the striking finding?

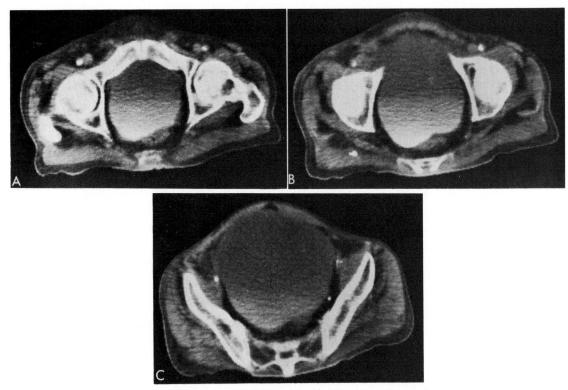

FIGURE 7–2a, b, c

The pelvic mass is clearly a distended urinary bladder. The urine opacified by contrast medium, which has a higher specific gravity than the nonopacified urine, is located in the dependent portion of the bladder. The rectum is seen behind the bladder and is compressed by it. The sigmoid colon and the small bowel normally seen in the pelvis have been displaced out of the pelvis by the distended bladder. Calcification in the arterial walls identifies the external iliac arteries at the medial margins of the iliopsoas muscles on section *c* and the femoral arteries ventral to the acetabula on sections *a* and *b*. In the mid-pelvic section there is a calcification in the right buttocks, probably an old injection site.

Mr. N. R. responds well to transurethral prostatic resection. There are certainly better ways to diagnose bladder outlet obstruction. In this patient CT excluded a significant mass, but other examinations will generally suffice.

Mr. C. P. is a 40 year old man who comes in with dysuria. He also has microscopic hematuria and the initial clinical impression is prostatitis. An intravenous urogram is obtained to look for other causes of hematuria. Do you see any abnormality?

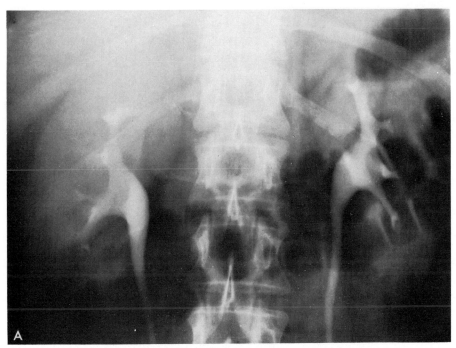

FIGURE 7–3a

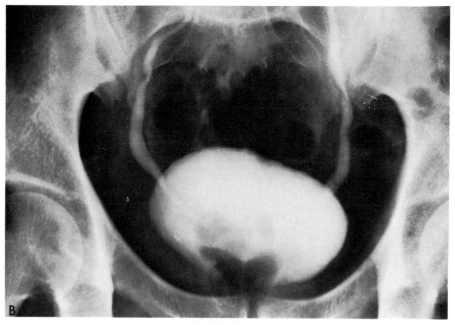

FIGURE 7–3b

The renal contours and collecting systems are normal. The bladder is also normal, though it is somewhat asymmetrical. Rectal gas is seen through the opacified bladder.

The patient next has cystoscopy, which reveals an extensive transitional cell carcinoma of the bladder. A CT examination is ordered to assist in staging the tumor.

The initial section was obtained at the level of the acetabula. A small amount of intravenous contrast medium has been given to opacify the bladder and ureters. What abnormalities do you see?

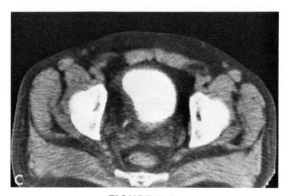

FIGURE 7–3c

Immediately anterior to the sacrum is the rectum with some fecal contents. The bow tie-shaped structure anterior to the rectum is the seminal vesicles. Anterior to this is the opacified bladder. The bladder is markedly abnormal, with thickening and irregularity of the right lateral and posterior portions of the bladder wall caused by extensive neoplastic infiltration. However, the fat planes between the bladder and the pelvic sidewalls are preserved bilaterally.

What do you make of the next section?

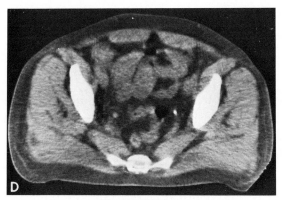

FIGURE 7–3d

Multiple loops of small bowel are present anteriorly. Posteriorly, the rectosigmoid colon is seen with some intraluminal gas. The ureters are seen bilaterally. There is no evidence of metastatic adenopathy. Since the disease is confined to the bladder, the carcinoma is treated surgically.

The staging of bladder carcinomas is facilitated by CT scanning. Bladder wall thickness is demonstrated and direct extravesical extension is well seen. Staging in the past has been difficult, since cystoscopy cannot evaluate transmural and extramural extension.

CASE 7–4:

MRS. E. P.

Mrs. E. P. is an elderly woman who had a total abdominal hysterectomy followed by pelvic irradiation for endometrial carcinoma ten years ago. She sees you for a routine checkup and you find microscopic hematuria. An intravenous urogram demonstrates moderate dilatation of the collecting systems bilaterally to the mid-pelvis but no masses are demonstrated. Cystoscopy reveals a transitional cell carcinoma of the bladder, which is infiltrating and poorly differentiated histologically. A CT scan is ordered in an attempt to differentiate tumor obstructing the distal ureters from radiation-induced fibrosis. Three sections are illustrated. The first was done before intravenous contrast material was given, though oral contrast medium has been given.

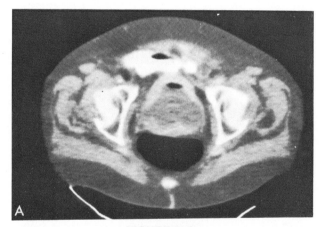

FIGURE 7–4a

The bladder is moderately distended with urine and the small amount of gas present was probably introduced during catheterization. The bladder wall is irregularly thickened ventrally but the fat planes around the bladder are intact. No tumor extension beyond the bladder is seen. The rectum is capacious and is distended with gas. Bowel loops are seen ventral to the bladder, a common finding when the bladder is not fully distended.

The next section shown was done after intravenous contrast material was given. The level is similar to the first section. What do you see?

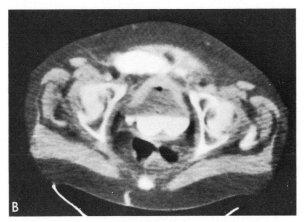

FIGURE 7–4b

The irregular bladder wall is again seen. The rectum has evacuated most of its gaseous content. Again no tumor extension is seen beyond the bladder wall. Scans covering the next 8 cm caphalad were all normal. The section at 10 cm cephalad is illustrated. What do you see?

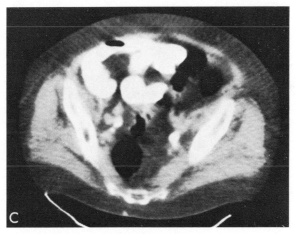

FIGURE 7–4c

The ureters are seen at this level and are quite dilated. There is no associated soft tissue mass. The absence of any soft tissue mass or dilated ureters between this level and the bladder makes you quite sure that the ureteral strictures are caused by radiation fibrosis from her earlier radiation therapy, and not extravesical tumor extension.

Mrs. E. P. responds well to local palliative therapy for her bladder tumor and her ureteral strictures do not progress during a year's followup. The role of CT scanning in this case is a negative one. The absence of masses and the preservation of normal tissue planes indicate that obstruction of the ureters by a malignancy is unlikely. Localization of the bladder carcinoma to the bladder wall made it possible to choose palliative local therapy for Mrs. E. P.

CASE 7–5:

MR. L. L.

Your patient Mr. L. L. is brought in by his niece, who cares for him. He is a cranky old fellow who rarely follows your advice. Now he complains that his "stream is off," and he is having trouble starting and stopping urination. On physical exam, he has a large lobular prostate. This time he is willing to accept hospitalization.

The consulting urologist feels a hard nodule, which he biopsies. This proves to be a carcinoma. Prior to definitive surgery, a CT scan is ordered to evaluate the pelvis for local extension. What do you see in the section at the level of the acetabular roof?

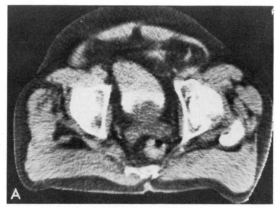

FIGURE 7–5a

The bladder is opacified by contrast medium. The enlarged median lobe of the prostate impresses the bladder base and the seminal vesicles are well seen dorsal to the prostate. The rectum and the pelvic fat planes are normal. Did you notice the ring-like structure on the left just beneath the abdominal muscles? This contains fat and some structures with higher attenuation. What do you think this is?

The next section is at the pubic symphysis. What is seen at this level?

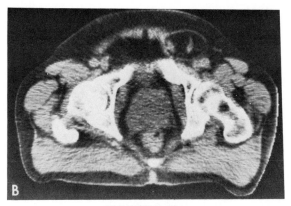

FIGURE 7–5b

The enlarged prostate is still seen. There is a bulge in its contour to the right, adjacent to the anterior aspect of the rectum. This is in the area of the clinically palpable nodule but it may represent asymmetric hypertrophy. It is not possible at present to tell malignant from adenomatous prostatic tissue by CT scan appearance. No evidence of extension of carcinoma is seen beyond the gland. Again, the ventral "ring" is seen. This time it lies between the rectus muscle and the femoral vessels. The next two sections are through the scrotum. The s-shaped structure is the corpus cavernosa of the penis. What do you see in the scrotum?

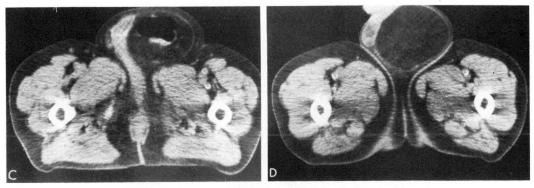

FIGURE 7–5c, d

The ring-like structure lies in the scrotum. In c, this is seen to contain a second ring, which has gas within it. It is clear that this is a large inguinal hernia containing both fat and bowel.

You have known about the hernia for many years. In fact, Mr. L. L. has refused to let you repair it. CT is certainly not the way to diagnose clinically obvious hernias, but this one is an interesting demonstration of the CT appearance of a hernia.

The report that the carcinoma seems to be confined to the prostate is good news, and Mr. L. L. decides to have surgery for both his prostatic difficulties and his inguinal hernia.

MR. S. K. AND MR. N. T.

Mr. S. K., a retired mechanic, has been hospitalized because of bladder outlet obstruction caused by an enlarged prostate. Before cystoscopy, a nodule is palpated in the prostate and a needle biopsy shows a well differentiated adenocarcinoma. Before deciding on therapy, you request a CT examination of the pelvis to be sure that the neoplasm is confined to the prostate. What do you see on this initial section through the level of the pubic symphysis? Intravenous contrast material has been given.

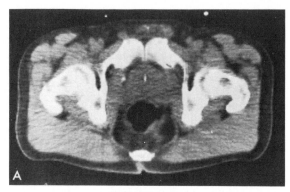

FIGURE 7–6a

The enlarged prostate lies behind the pubic symphysis. There is a high attenuation dot in its center. This is urine opacified by contrast medium in the lumen of the Foley catheter. It locates the urethra and shows the relationship of the prostate to the urethra. Behind the prostate is the rectum, distended with gas. It is separated from the prostate by a thin fat plane. Lateral and posterior to the rectum is the normal fat and connective tissue of the pelvis. What about the next section 1 cm more cranial?

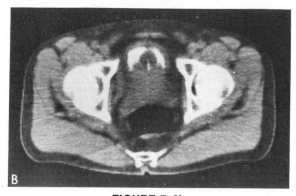

FIGURE 7–6b

The section shows the thickened bladder wall and the balloon of the Foley catheter with opacified urine around it and in the catheter lumen. The enlarged median lobe bulges into the dorsal aspect of the bladder. Posterolateral to the prostate are the seminal vesicles. The rectum is still distended with gas. The next section is slightly higher. What do you make of this?

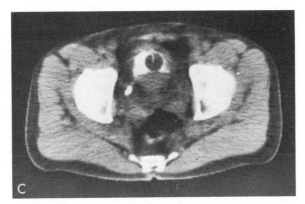

FIGURE 7–6c

The large median lobe is again seen impressing the posterior aspect of the bladder. This is the usual appearance of benign prostatic hypertrophy. No evidence of tumor spread is demonstrated on these sections and Mr. S. K.'s prostatic carcinoma is not visualized. At present it is not possible to detect intraglandular malignant tissue by CT scanning. The important information gained is the absence of abnormal tissue beyond the prostate, the presence of which would indicate pelvic spread.

The large median lobe is confirmed at surgery. Mr. S. K. makes a rapid recovery and is soon working in his garden again.

Mr. N. T.'s is a similar story but his CT scan has a more striking abnormality. What do you think of this section?

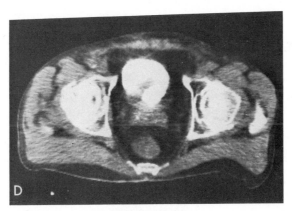

FIGURE 7–6d

There is an angular finger-like projection of soft tissue sticking into the opacified bladder. It is tempting to think that this apparent projection into the bladder is a tumor arising from the bladder mucosa. Look at the film of the bladder from the intravenous urogram on the next page. Does this help to explain what you are seeing?

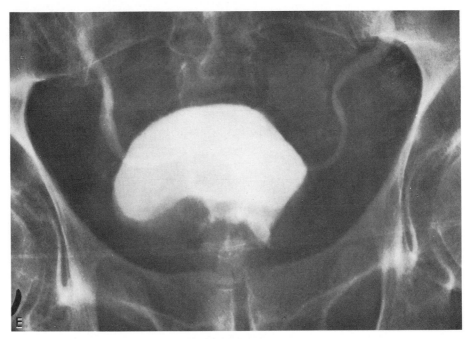

FIGURE 7–6e

There is a markedly lobulated impression on the base of the bladder. This is caused by enlargement in the median lobe of the prostate. When these lobulations are sectioned in the transaxial plane, they are seen as ridges of soft tissue. At cystoscopy, no tumor is present in the bladder and the bladder mucosa is intact and normal.

Great care must be taken in interpreting scans at the bladder base, since asymmetric prostatic enlargement can produce mass-like excrescences that appear to be intravesicular on both CT and conventional cystograms.

Mr. A. L. is a 48 year old man who is referred to you for acute urinary retention. His internist has felt a large prostate but cannot pass a catheter. You do manage to catheterize the patient and when his acute distress is alleviated, you obtain a more complete history. Mr. A. L. has not really been feeling well for several months and has lost about 20 pounds. He runs daily but has cut his distance from 5 to about 2 miles a day because of fatigue. His urinary stream has been diminishing for some time but he has paid little attention to this. Your physical examination confirms the enlarged prostate, which is hard and knobby. The abdomen feels full. Intravenous urogram shows only the enlarged prostate and abdominal ultrasound is unsatisfactory because of bowel gas. When a prostatic needle biopsy reveals anaplastic carcinoma, you order a CT scan for assistance in staging the carcinoma. The scan is performed after the intravenous injection of 20 cc of contrast medium. The pelvis and the abdomen are examined. Two scans of contiguous pelvic areas are demonstrated. What do you see?

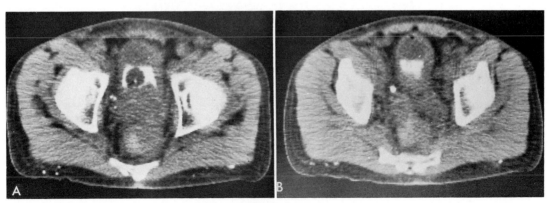

FIGURE 7–7a, b

The balloon of the Foley catheter is seen surrounded by contrast material. A bulky mass deforms the posterior bladder wall. This is the prostate enlarged by carcinoma. There are enlarged left inguinal nodes. Section *b* shows a small amount of air in the dome of the bladder as well as a fluid-fluid level caused by urine and contrast medium. The enlarged prostate is again seen dorsal to the bladder. The right ureter is seen filled with contrast material. Small bowel loops are present in the pelvis, but there is also abnormal soft tissue dorsal and lateral to the bladder and prostate.

The upper two sections are through the mid and lower abdomen. What do you see on the lower section?

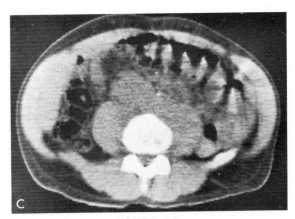

FIGURE 7–7c

The tip of the right lobe of the liver is seen. Normal colon and small bowel fill the abdominal cavity. The retroperitoneum is markedly abnormal. The aorta and the inferior vena cava are engulfed by a soft tissue mass that has obliterated all the usual fat planes. The mass extends laterally over the psoas muscles. This appearance is typical of massive adenopathy. Now look at the higher section.

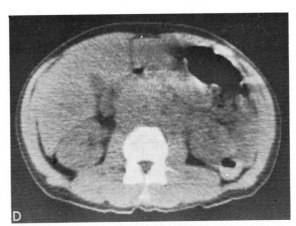

FIGURE 7–7d

The kidneys, the right lobe of the liver and the gallbladder are all seen on this section. The aorta and the inferior vena cava are again shown engulfed by enlarged nodes.

The massive extent of Mr. A. L.'s tumor surprises you. His therapy is modified markedly, since local pelvic radiation obviously will not control his disease.

In the past, lymphography would have been needed to stage Mr. A. L.'s disease. Lymphography can be misleading about the full extent of adenopathy, since lymphatic channels may be obstructed, replaced nodes may not fill at all and nodes above the cisterna chyli are not demonstrated.

Mr. A. L. does only moderately well on systemic chemotherapy and after about six months the decision is made to place him on another drug protocol. Before starting the new regimen, you request a repeat CT scan as a baseline for tumor response. He has been complaining of constipation, so you also order a barium enema. Though it is done after the CT scan, you can study it first. The film demonstrated is a lateral spot film of the rectosigmoid colon. What do you see?

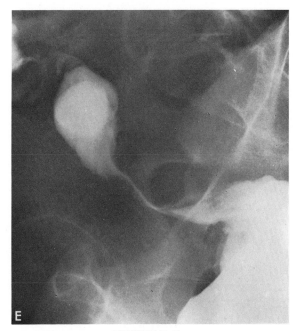

FIGURE 7-7e

The colon is markedly narrowed and there is significant increase in the soft tissues between the colon and the sacrum. The narrowing appears to be extrinsic on all films of the rectum and sigmoid colon. The narrowing explains the constipation but is somewhat unusual in prostate carcinoma. You review the CT scan, which was done after both oral and intravenous contrast media have been given. What observations do you make on the first section?

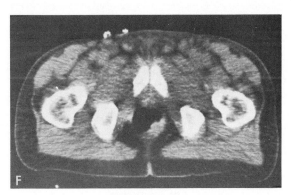

FIGURE 7-7f

This scan is done at the pubic symphysis. Bilateral inguinal adenopathy is seen at this time. The most interesting finding is the irregularity and asymmetry of the rectum, which is thickened on the left. The next section is higher in the pelvis. What do you see here?

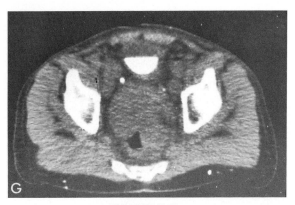

FIGURE 7–7g

A fluid-fluid level is seen in the bladder. Node masses are present bilaterally. The prostate has enlarged even more and is engulfing the rectum, displacing it to the right and somewhat ventrally. This correlates very well with the barium enema findings. The final section shown is in mid-abdomen. What do you make of it?

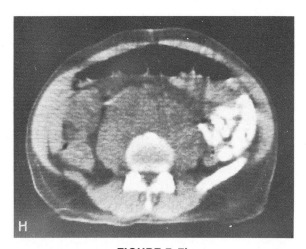

FIGURE 7–7h

The massive prevertebral adenopathy is still present and has probably increased in size since the study done seven months earlier.

The volume of tumor seems overwhelming to you but Mr. A. L. is a born fighter. After discussing the alternatives with his family, he decides to try the new drug protocol. His initial response is encouraging and you plan to follow his case with limited CT scans.

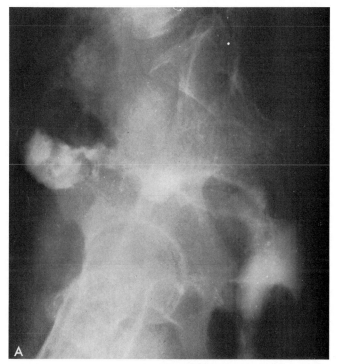

MR. O. M.

Mr. O. M., a frail, elderly gentleman who has been your patient for many years, complains of constipation and difficulty urinating. On physical examination you feel a lobular mass in the anterolateral aspect of the rectum, which you think is probably prostatic in origin. However, there is also nodularity posteriorly in the rectum that greatly concerns you. Sigmoidoscopy is attempted, but the instrument can be passed only a few centimeters into the rectum before the advance is blocked by an encircling mass. A barium enema is ordered. What do you see?

FIGURE 7–8a

There is a long abnormal segment with both anterior and posterior nodularity and mucosal destruction. The radiologist thinks that primary carcinoma of the rectum is the most likely diagnosis, though extensive infiltration from prostatic carcinoma could have this appearance. You decide to order a CT scan to try to assess the extent of the disease and to evaluate the prostate. What do you think of the first section through the pubic symphysis?

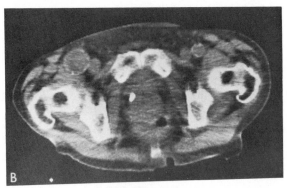

FIGURE 7–8b

The prostate is enlarged in a rather lobular fashion. The rectal wall seems very thick and the rectal gas is markedly asymmetric. Lateral to the rectum the tissue planes are preserved. Did you see anything else? You should have noticed that calcification is present in the femoral arteries and that the right femoral artery is aneurysmal. What about the next section through the bladder base? The bladder has been opacified by intravenous contrast.

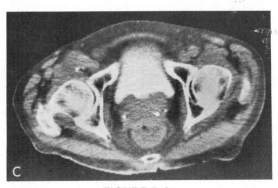

FIGURE 7–8c

The contrast-filled bladder has a prominent bilobed prostatic impression posteriorly. There are calcifications within and adjacent to the prostate that are probably phleboliths. The fat lateral to the bladder and prostate is normal. The rectum contains little gas and is filled with soft tissue. Stool can be confusing in the rectum, but in this case we know that the rectal lumen is encircled. The fat between the rectum and the levator sling is intact anteriorly. There is a thin crescent of lucency separating the rectal mass from the enlarged prostate. The next section is through the lower abdomen. Is any information added? Oral contrast material has been given.

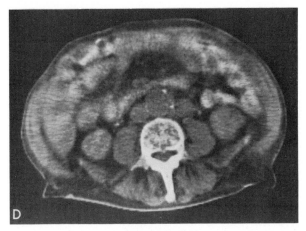

FIGURE–8d

The important observation lies in the retroperitoneum. The aorta is aneurysmal and to its right is the inferior vena cava. On the left of the aorta is an enlarged lymph node. This is metastatic disease extending beyond the pelvis.

The findings are those of rectal carcinoma with extension to distant nodes. For this reason radical surgery is abandoned, and diverting colostomy, transurethral prostatectomy and radiation therapy are employed. Although Mr. O. M. does not survive for long, he is comfortable. You are glad that he has been spared unnecessary surgery.

CASE 7–9:

MR. B. K.

Mr. B. K. is a 60 year old man who had an abdominoperineal resection for a cloacogenic carcinoma of the rectum one year ago. Initially he did well, but now he has developed deep pelvic pain and tenderness over the sacroiliac joints. Radiographs of the pelvis are taken to look for bony metastases. Do you see any abnormality?

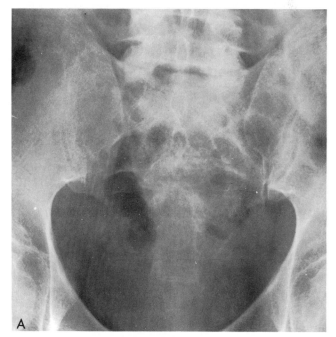

FIGURE 7–9a

The films of the pelvis are not definitely abnormal, though the left sacral wing is indistinct and so a radionuclide bone scan is obtained. The posterior whole body view is shown. What do you see?

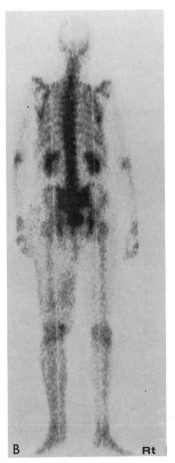

FIGURE 7–9b

An area of intense uptake of radioisotope is confined to the sacrum. No other bony abnormalities are seen. The radionuclide is also present in the kidneys and the urinary bladder. The symptoms and isotopic findings suggest a local tumor recurrence and a CT scan is obtained to further evaluate the soft tissues of the pelvis. The initial scan is just above the pubic symphysis. What structures are seen?

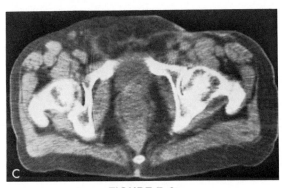

FIGURE 7–9c

The prostate is immediately behind the pubic rami. In the normal patient the rectum lies behind the prostate, but this patient has had an abdominoperineal resection and has no rectum. While surgical scar can account for a portion of this soft tissue, tumor recurrence is quite likely. The fat and muscles of the pelvic side walls are intact.

A section through the acetabula also shows an abnormal soft tissue mass immediately anterior to the sacrum.

The next section illustrated is cephalad to the bladder at the mid-sacrum. Here the abnormalities are more marked.

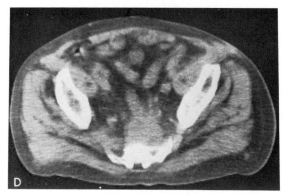

FIGURE 7–9d

There is a bulky, lobular soft tissue mass anterior to the sacrum. No fat plane separates the mass from the sacrum and the anterior aspect of the sacrum is destroyed. This is particularly obvious on the right.

The next section is through the sacroiliac joints. Both ureters are filled with contrast material.

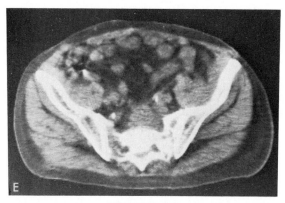

FIGURE 7–9e

In this section, the lobular mass again straddles the midline and invades the anterior sacral cortex. The left ureter is displaced anteriorly by the mass.

The findings are those of an extensive local recurrence of carcinoma, extending from the pelvic floor to the top of the sacrum, with some destruction of the sacrum. The patient is treated with local radiotherapy for palliation of pain.

While bony destruction is often well seen at CT scanning, radionuclide studies have a much greater sensitivity and radiographs show more detail. Slight variations in the patient positioning can suggest bony erosion during CT scanning by producing an asymmetrical partial volume effect. Setting with window width and mean for optimum viewing of the bones in question should also be done when bony erosion comes into question.

Your patient, Mrs. M. M., is found to have lymphoma on a biopsy of an enlarged cervical node. An abdominal CT scan is obtained to help in staging the lymphoma. During the examination an unrelated abnormality is discovered in the pelvis. What is it? Intravenous contrast has been given.

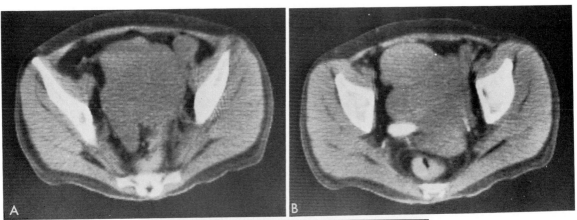

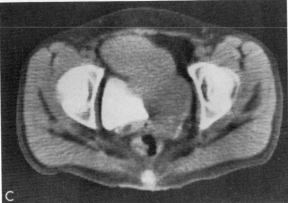

FIGURE 7–10a, b, c

On section *a* there is a large lobulated mass that displaces bowel. On section *b*, a bit of the contrast filled bladder and both ureters are seen. The large lobular mass fills the middle of the pelvis. A portion of the mass lies between the bladder and the rectum, compressing the rectum. The bulk of the mass is anterior and superior to the bladder. On the last section, the bladder is displaced to the right. The lobulated mass extends ventrally and to the right. The mass is very homogeneous and has an attenuation similar to muscle. The homogeneous nature of the mass and the lobulated contour suggest a myomatous uterus.

Most pelvic masses should be studied by ultrasound. The needed information is generally obtained and no radiation is used. CT should be reserved for situations in which ultrasound does not or cannot provide the answers desired. The CT appearance of leiomyomata is generally that seen here. However, if hemorrhage, necrosis or calcification have occurred, the mass will be inhomogeneous.

CASE 7–11:

MRS. B. R.

   Mrs. B. R. is a 53 year old woman who had total hysterectomy for a Stage II carcinoma of the cervix about three years ago. She has been well until quite recently, when she developed some dull, rather diffuse lower back pain. It does not go away and she calls you for advice. She has always been a reliable observer of her physical status, so you ask her to come in for a checkup. Pelvic examination reveals a diffuse fullness, but you cannot identify a discrete mass. You order an intravenous urogram and barium enema to try to better define the problem. The abnormalities on the urogram are a surprise but do provide an explanation for her symptoms. What do you see on the two films?

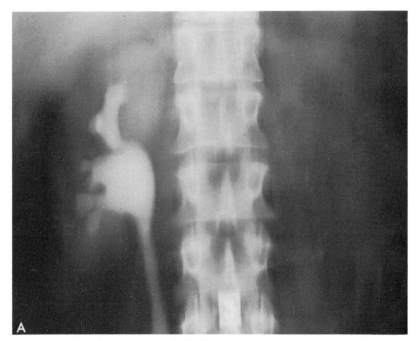

FIGURE 7–11a

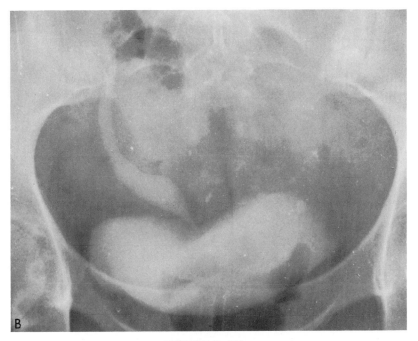

FIGURE 7–11b

The left kidney does not function and there is dilatation of the collecting system on the right. A mass displaces the bladder.

Barium enema is done immediately following the intravenous urogram and one film is shown. What does it tell you?

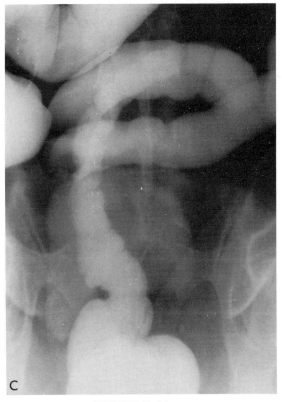

FIGURE 7–11c

The film is an angled view of the distal sigmoid colon and rectum. In Mrs. B. R., the sigmoid colon is straightened and lifted out of the pelvis by a large mass. The bladder still has some contrast medium in it.

Mrs. B. R. seems to have an extensive recurrence of her cervical carcinoma and radiation therapy is considered. The alternatives are radical surgery or chemotherapy and radiation for palliation. You order a CT scan to accurately evaluate tumor extent. What do you see on these sections? Intravenous contrast material has been given.

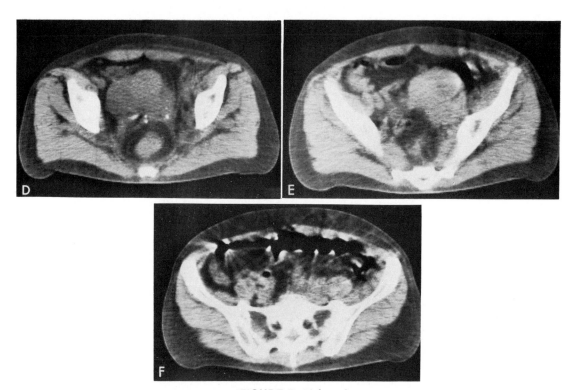

FIGURE 7–11d, e, f

Section *d* performed at about 3 cm above the symphysis shows a lobular mass engulfing the bladder, which is faintly opacified with contrast material. There are enlarged lymph nodes along the left pelvic side wall. The next section, 3 cm higher, continues to show left pelvic wall adenopathy and the large tumor mass. Section *f* has extensive artifacts caused by peristalsis and colon gas. Left prevertebral adenopathy is demonstrated.

The urinary tract obstruction is the most pressing aspect of Mrs. B. R.'s tumor recurrence. Surgical intervention is considered, but the patient prefers to have a trial of combined radiation and chemotherapy.

Mrs. Z. B. returns for a routine followup visit. She has felt well for most of the eight months since her total abdominal hysterectomy and oophorectomy for ovarian cystadenocarcinoma. Now, however, she complains of a "dragging" pain in the pelvis. Physical examination reveals a bulky mass in the mid-pelvis and an ultrasound is ordered. What do you see in this transverse section of the pelvis?

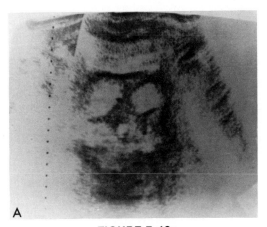

FIGURE 7-12a

The bladder contains many echoes, which are artifactual. Behind the bladder there is a large complex mass with areas of high and low echogenicity typical of fluid and solid components. This ultrasound picture is quite compatible with recurrent cystadenocarcinoma. You decide to get an intravenous urogram to evaluate renal function and ureteric involvement by the mass. Is any information added on the ten minute full film of the abdomen?

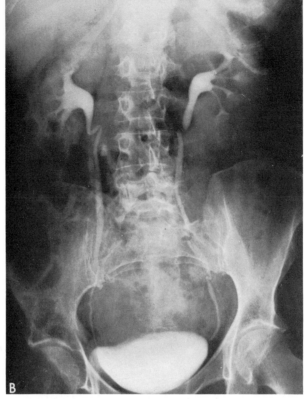

FIGURE 7–12b

There is a large soft tissue mass in the pelvis that deviates the ureters laterally but no obstruction is present. There is no other abnormality on this film, but review the coned-down view of the kidneys.

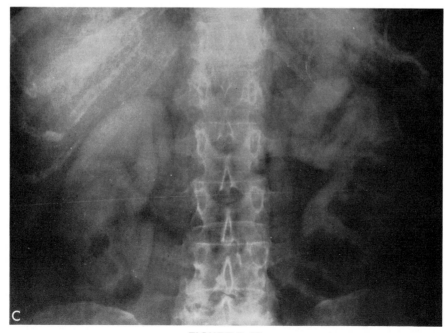

FIGURE 7–12c

The axis of the left kidney seems more vertical than normal. There is also the suggestion of a soft tissue mass superimposed on the left upper pole. Because of these suggestive findings you order a CT scan to more completely assess the extent of disease. The initial section illustrated is through the pelvis. Intravenous contrast material has been given. Does this confirm the sonographic findings?

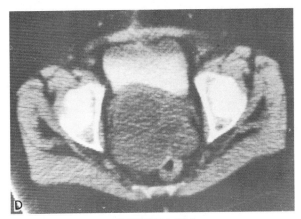

FIGURE 7–12d

There is a large mass interposed between the rectum and the bladder. The round areas of lower attenuation are the fluid-containing areas seen on the sonogram. The correlation with the sonogram is good and the muscular and bony structures of the pelvis are better visualized.

The next section is above the true pelvis. Oral contrast material has been given. Is there any abnormality?

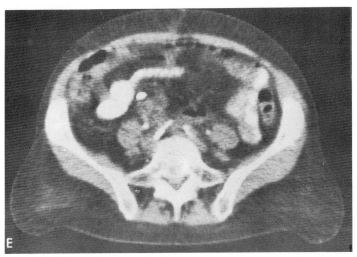

FIGURE 7–12e

The findings here are subtle. The ureters are opacified bilaterally and are in normal position adjacent to the psoas muscles. Anterior to the right ureter there is a small oval collection of contrast medium in bowel, but the soft tissue between these two structures is metastatic adenopathy.

Look at the next sections, through the left kidney. Do these help to explain the urographic findings?

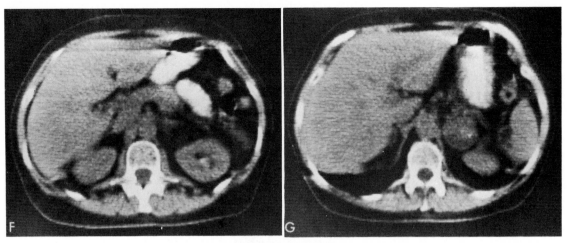

FIGURE 7–12f, g

On section *f* the kidney appears normal. The inferior aspect of the left adrenal gland is seen lateral to the aorta and dorsal to the pancreas, and it is slightly enlarged. On section *g* 2 cm cephalad there is an obvious mass lateral to the aorta, medial to the upper pole of the left kidney and dorsal to the splenic vein. This mass has high and low attenuation areas that are similar to the CT appearance of the primary ovarian cystadenocarcinoma. The mass is a metastasis to the left adrenal gland.

Because of the presence of metastatic disease beyond the pelvis, consideration of further surgery or radiotherapy is dropped and Mrs. Z. B. is placed on chemotherapy. Her initial response is good and so her spirits are high when she leaves town for the opera season at Glyndebourne.

MR. B. G. AND MR. J. B.

Mr. B. G. is a 58 year old former wrestler who has to be admitted to the hospital because of acute urinary retention. Physical examination shows some prostatic enlargement. After the patient is catheterized, you order an intravenous urogram. What do you see on the ten minute film?

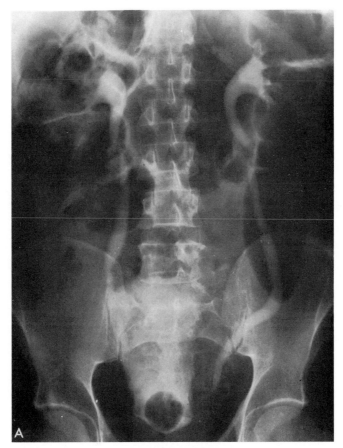

FIGURE 7–13a

Both ureters are somewhat distended. The bladder is elevated and has an unusual pear-shaped configuration. There are multiple lobular impressions on the bladder, especially laterally. Below the bladder is a vague rounded soft tissue density that is the prostate, but why is it seen at all?

The diffuse lucency around the bladder and throughout the pelvis suggests pelvic lipomatosis, but there are other causes for bilateral irregular impressions on the bladder. You decide to order a CT scan to confirm the diagnosis of pelvic lipomatosis. What do you make of this first section?

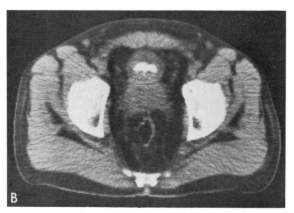

FIGURE 7–13b

Contrast medium is seen in the base of the bladder. The enlarged prostate lies behind the bladder. Gas identifies the rectum, which is surrounded by an unusual amount of fat. The next two sections are higher in the pelvis. What do you see?

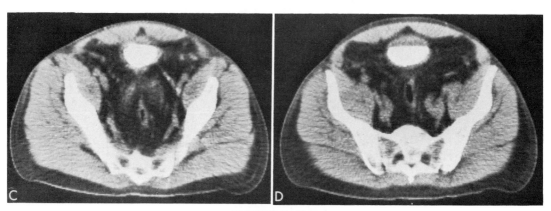

FIGURE 7–13c, d

The bladder wall appears thickened. The rectosigmoid colon is compressed into a slit by the markedly increased pelvic fat. The diagnosis of pelvic lipomatosis is confirmed and other more serious pelvic masses are excluded. Mr. B. G. has a good response to transurethral prostatic resection.

This case demonstrates the utility of CT in pelvic lipomatosis because of the ability to accurately measure tissue x-ray attenuation.

Shortly after Mr. B. G. is discharged from the hospital, Mr. J. B., a 30 year old stocky black, comes to your office complaining of a one year history of urinary frequency and pain on urination. He has been told by several doctors that he has prostatitis or cystitis and has been treated with antibiotics to no avail. Physical examination reveals only an elevated blood pressure. Mr. J. B. says he has had high blood pressure for "a while," and he has been taking pills. You need to investigate both the lower urinary tract complaints and the hypertension, so you request an intravenous urogram. The upper urinary tracts are normal. What do you see on this post voiding film of the pelvis and the bladder?

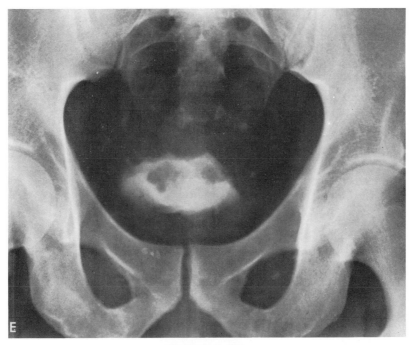

FIGURE 7–13e

The bladder is elevated from the pelvic floor; the wall appears too thickened and irregular even for a contracted bladder. The tissues around the bladder are also abnormally lucent.

Since the urologic problem seems to be localized to the lower urinary tract, cystoscopy is performed. This examination is difficult because of elongation of the bladder neck. The bladder wall is rigid and a biopsy reveals chronic inflammation.

The radiologist and the consulting urologist think that the most likely diagnosis is pelvic lipomatosis. A CT scan is requested to confirm this diagnosis. The first scan is through the bladder base. Is any information added?

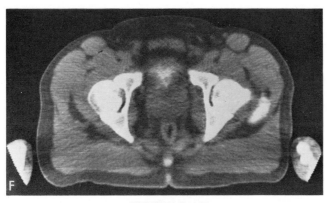

FIGURE 7–13f

The irregular thickened bladder base is seen. Between the bladder base and the rectum is a soft tissue density, an enlarged prostate. The next section is 2 cm cephalad. The bladder is better distended. Is any other structure abnormal?

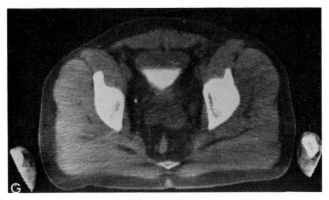

FIGURE 7–13g

The superior aspect of the prostate is again seen behind the bladder. Behind this are seminal vesicles, enlarged particularly on the left. There is a diffuse moderate increase in pelvic fat. The next section is more cranial and the findings even more striking. What do you see?

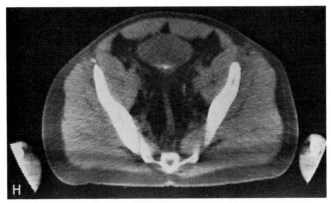

FIGURE 7–13h

Behind the bladder there is a thin structure running back to the sacrum. This is the markedly compressed sigmoid colon. The remainder of the pelvis is filled with increased pelvic fat, which displaces small bowel out of the pelvis and compresses the sigmoid colon. These findings confirm the urographic diagnosis of pelvic lipomatosis.

It is not known whether the pelvic lipomatosis is a response to or the cause of chronic lower urinary tract inflammation. The condition may progress to complete ureteral obstruction, a condition requiring a urinary diversion. Young black males are particularly prone to this severe form of pelvic lipomatosis. Mr. J. B. is placed on long term antibiotic therapy for cystitis and prostatitis and on antihypertensive medication. The seriousness of his problems are stressed and he agrees to close followup.

Mr. R. W. is a charming elderly gentleman who underwent surgery and then radiation therapy for prostatic carcinoma about one year ago. He makes no complaints on a routine followup visit, but you palpate a definite left lower quadrant mass and wonder about a second one on the right. Your probing causes some discomfort. Close questioning finally elicits a history of some weight loss and increased fatigue. You decide to order an abdominal film and an ultrasound to be followed by CT scan, intravenous urography or barium studies as needed.

The abdominal film demonstrates a left lower quadrant mass but does not aid in its diagnosis. Ultrasound is limited by bowel contents but does demonstrate two masses. The one on the right is smaller than the one on the left. The masses have a fluid component but good definition of the wall is not obtained.

The fluid nature of the masses raises the question of bilateral lymphoceles following the node dissection and recurrent tumor seems less likely. It seems unlikely that barium studies or even intravenous urography will add much useful information, so you request a CT scan. The patient has been given water soluble oral contrast medium prior to scanning. Two sections are demonstrated. What are your observations?

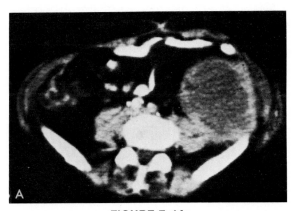

FIGURE 7–14a

The first section shows a large round mass in the left lower abdomen. It has a thick irregular wall and a central area of decreased attenuation. Bowel is displaced by the mass and the peritoneum is thickened lateral to the mass.

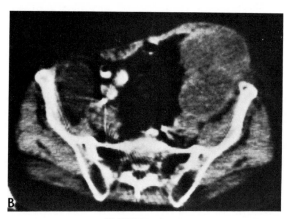

FIGURE 7–14b

The second scan shows septations in the left mass and demonstrates a similar, though much smaller, mass on the right. The extensive bowel gas on both cuts explains why the ultrasound was only partially successful; the gas also has caused artifacts on the CT scans. Mr. R. W. and his CT scan don't fit together well because the irregular thick walls of the masses make lymphoceles unlikely. On the other hand, he seems too well to have abscesses or massive necrotic tumor, which the CT findings suggest.

When you discuss your diagnostic dilemma with Mr. R. W., he mentions running an occasional low grade fever. You decide on a limited laparotomy for biopsy or drainage and are rather pleased to find two abscesses. Purulent material from the abscesses later grows *E. coli*. It is never clear why Mr. R. W. got his abscesses, but his course is benign and he leaves the hospital eight days after drainage.

Mrs. F. L. returns to your office complaining of increasing right hip pain. Two years ago she had similar complaints about the left hip, and evaluation revealed avascular necrosis of the left femoral head that was treated successfully by total hip replacement. You send Mrs. F. L. for radiographs of the right hip and pelvis. What do you see?

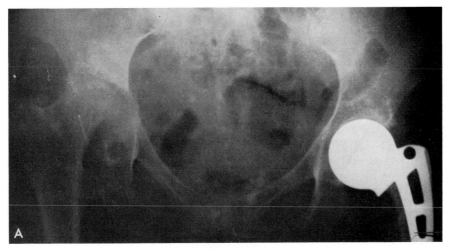

FIGURE 7–15a

The left total hip prosthesis is in a proper position and has caused little reaction. On the right, there are now changes of advanced avascular necrosis with destruction of the femoral head. This surprises you because Mrs. F. L. insists that her right hip has hurt for only two weeks. Closer scrutiny of the film reveals displacement of the phleboliths along the right pelvic side wall toward the midline. Compare the right-sided phleboliths with the more normally positioned phleboliths on the left. This suggests a mass along the right pelvic side wall.

You are concerned about this finding and question Mrs. F. L. more closely. She admits that she has had some malaise and has thought she had fever, but she has been preoccupied with her pain and inability to get around. Tumor and aneurysm are two possible causes of the mass. A CT scan is ordered to try to get a better idea of what is going on. What do you make of this first section?

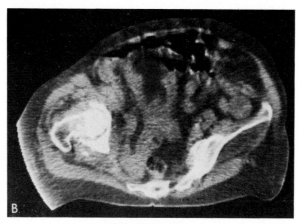

FIGURE 7-15b

The most remarkable thing about this section is the asymmetry of the bony pelvis. The left side of the section is through the iliac crest and the right is through the acetabulum. What do you suppose has caused this?

The patient has been placed in the scanning gantry at an angle to keep the plane of the section on the left above the metallic hip prosthesis. The prosthesis would generate extensive artifacts, obscuring all the soft tissues in the pelvis.

The bony wall of the right acetabulum is intact, though the joint space and femoral head are abnormal. The soft tissue that is seen in the pelvis at this level is all small bowel and colon. What do you think of the next section, which is 2 cm more inferior? Intravenous contrast medium has been given to opacify the bladder.

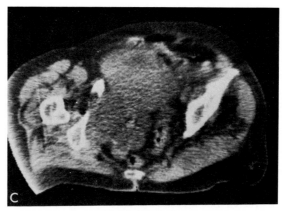

FIGURE 7-15c

There is a lobulated soft tissue mass behind and to the right of the faintly opacified bladder. The mass impresses the right posterolateral aspect of the bladder. It is not in continuity with the rectosigmoid seen in the left pelvis nor does it extend through the obturator foramen into the thigh. Internally the mass is rather homogeneous, with lower attenuation than muscle, but it contains no fat or gas.

The mass itself is nonspecific in appearance, but because of the absence of abdominal symptoms and the mild systemic symptoms, lymphoma is favored as the preoperative diagnosis. At surgery, however, the mass is found to be an abscess caused by an appendiceal rupture. Without the presence of gas or a gas-fluid level within the lesion, this diagnosis cannot be made on the basis of the CT scans alone. Aspiration of the right hip does not produce purulent material. After drainage of the abscess, the hip pain disappears. The planned hip surgery is deferred.

You may wonder why ultrasound of the pelvis was not performed, since it is an excellent diagnostic modality in the pelvis. The reason CT was performed first is the very lateral position of the mass. Lesions along the bony pelvic side walls are very difficult to evaluate with ultrasound.

CASE 7–16:

MRS. C. M.

Your patient, Mrs. C. M., returns for a routine visit. She is a 45 year old housewife with lymphoma diagnosed by cervical node biopsy. Her initial evaluation showed mediastinal and upper abdominal adenopathy, but she had a good response to chemotherapy and has been relatively well for 18 months. Now she tires easily and you feel a lump in her right groin. You fear that Mrs. C. M.'s lymphoma is becoming more active and order a CT scan to assess the extent of disease. What do you make of the first section just above the pubic symphysis? Intravenous contrast has been given.

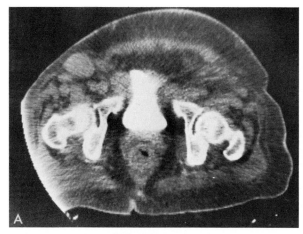

FIGURE 7–16a

The bladder is opacified by contrast medium. Behind the bladder are the uterus and rectum. The pelvic fat and muscle appear normal. On the right, anterior to the femoral head, there is a group of enlarged nodes, one of which is massive. Note the artifact generated by the patient's thigh, which was in contact with the scanning gantry. What do you see on the next section through the acetabula?

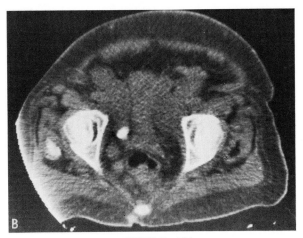

FIGURE 7-16b

The external iliac nodes are markedly enlarged and lobular. The uterus is anteverted and lies sandwiched between the nodal masses. A small amount of contrast material is seen on the right in the dome of the bladder. The rectum contains some gas. Did you notice the line of round soft tissue structures in the fat lateral to the rectum on the right? These are enlarged hypogastric lymph nodes. There are some just posterior and to the left of the rectum as well. What do you make of the next section? This is above the umbilicus, through the kidneys. Oral contrast medium is present in the stomach.

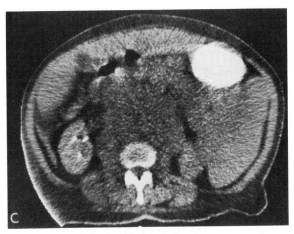

FIGURE 7-16c

There is extensive disease at this level as well. The enlarged para-aortic nodes form a mantle that obscures the aorta and inferior vena cava. The spleen is enlarged, and a poorly defined lobular mass of nodes fills the splenic hilum.

You are not surprised that Mrs. C. M. has recurrent disease. However, the extent and bulk of the adenopathy, including very extensive pelvic adenopathy, is unexpected. After discussion with the patient and consultation with other physicians, it is decided to try Mrs. C. M. on an experimental drug protocol at another institution. You do not see her again.

CHAPTER
8

CT OF THE CHEST

Intrathoracic pathology can be adequately defined by conventional chest radiographs and tomography in the vast majority of clinical situations. In the few situations in which CT has a place, a successful examination depends on the ability of the patient to suspend respiration for the duration of each scan, since breathing causes gross motion of all the thoracic structures. Even if respiration is completely eliminated, cardiac motion always degrades the image. Future instruments with faster scanning times or gating the scanning to the EKG may overcome this limitation and make transaxial cardiac scanning a more practical reality.

The advantages of CT in the chest are similar to those in other areas. The unique transaxial sections provided by CT demonstrate the relationship of one structure to another in the chest. For example, knowing the relationship of a lung mass to the mediastinum or of mediastinal masses to the great vessels can be useful to the surgeon. Intravenous contrast material may be injected to define the great vessels and to demonstrate vascular abnormalities such as aneurysms.

The increased sensitivity of CT to differences in tissue attenuation make it possible to identify fatty masses such as lipomas and structures of fluid density such as cysts and fissural "pseudotumors." Pleural fluid collections may be identified and localized for aspiration. The ability to examine the subpleural lung and the pulmonary recesses means that small occult metastases that are not demonstrated by conventional tomograms may be identified by CT.

As always, the CT examination must be designed to fit the clinical situation and the information desired. The number of sections, the scanning interval and the use of contrast material will vary from case to case. Conventional chest radiographs are an invaluable aid in planning a study and should always be available for review.

NORMAL CHEST AND VARIATIONS

The CT examination of the chest can be displayed in several ways, which are chosen to provide the most information about the structure in question. Some of the sections illustrated here will be shown both in the conventional technique and in a technique using a very low mean to demonstrate small structures in the lung itself. The CT examination of the chest differs from the conventional chest radiograph in that the examination is performed with the patient supine, though prone or decubitus views may also be obtained. Normal anatomy and variations must be kept in mind during the examination and while interpreting the scans.

The first scans illustrated are from an examination of a young man. They were made at the level of the aortic arch. What structures do you see?

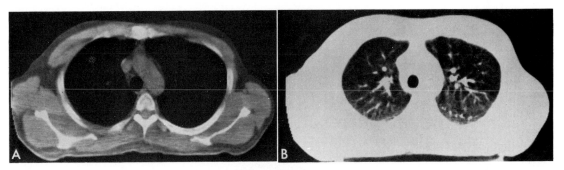

FIGURE 8–1a, b

Compare the lung detail seen on conventional scan *a* with that on the low mean scan *b*. You can easily identify the pulmonary vessels on *b*; no pulmonary detail is seen on *a*. The round, very low attenuation structure in the mediastinum is the trachea. The transverse portion of the aorta is seen as an oval extending from the anterior to posterior on scan *a*. Mediastinal fat is seen at the lateral and anterior aspects of the aortic arch. Adjacent to the anterior aspect of the arch is a round structure, the superior vena cava. Anterior to the aortic arch at this level, the lungs are separated by a considerable amount of soft tissue. The thymus is located in this area but is not seen as a separate structure. The next sections are just below the carina. What structures can you identify?

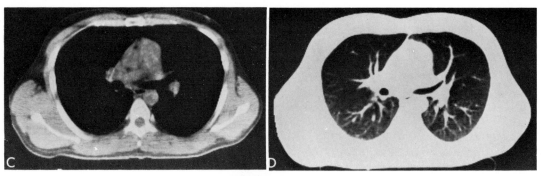

FIGURE 8–1c, d

The mainstem bronchi are the air-containing tubes extending into the pulmonary roots. The more horizontally oriented left mainstem bronchus is seen over a longer extent. The esophagus also contains air and lies behind the proximal left mainstem bronchus. It is best seen on section *c*. Adjacent to the esophagus is the descending aorta. Just to the right and behind the esophagus is the azygous vein. The right lung extends behind the right main bronchus toward the midline, forming the azygoesophageal recess of the right lung. Anterior to the bronchi are the cardiac outflow tracts. The ascending aorta is on the right and the main pulmonary artery is on the left. The main pulmonary artery is seen to divide, its right branch passing transversely behind the aorta to reach the right hilum and the left branch rapidly entering the left hilum to arborize in the lung. The right and left pleura are very closely opposed in their anterior aspect.

The next section was through the heart. Cardiac motion caused some artifact. What do you see?

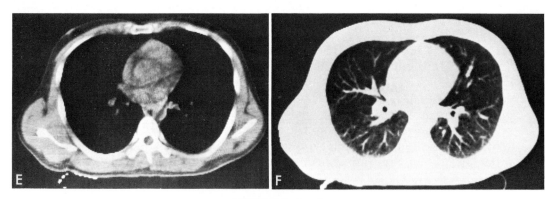

FIGURE 8–1e, f

The blood-filled cardiac chambers are seen on section *e*. There is some air in the esophagus adjacent to the descending aorta. The anterior mediastinum is very thin. The lung is not separated from the chest wall, since the normal pleura is not identified at CT scanning. Pleural fluid collections and thickenings or masses, both free and loculated, will separate the lung from the chest wall and will be seen at CT scanning.

The next scan is an upper chest section of an older man. Does anything strike your eye?

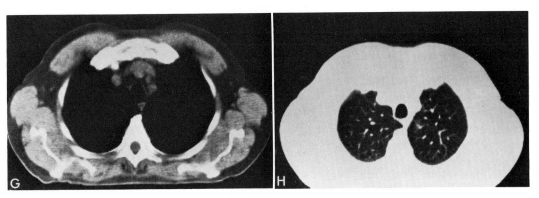

FIGURE 8–1g, h

There is a prominent rightward bulge in the anterior mediastinum. This is caused by tortuosity of the brachiocephalic vessels and should not be confused with a significant mass. If there is a question, intravenous contrast material may be used to opacify vessels.

What about the next sections through the heart?

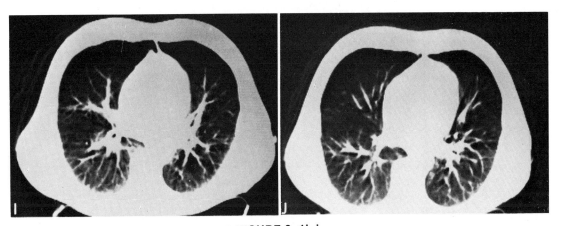

FIGURE 8–1i, j

These sections have been displayed at a very low mean to enhance soft tissue detail in the lung itself. Notice how deeply the right lung extends into the midline behind the right hilum. The gravitational distribution of blood flow to dependent portions of the lung is well seen. This phenomenon accounts for the increased x-ray attenuation posteriorly in the dependent lung; this should not be confused with a disease process.

The mode of display used for thoracic scan will determine the type of information available for interpretation. The examples you have just studied should emphasize this point. Standard body display will allow evaluation of the mediastinum and the chest wall. A display with a very low mean is needed for evaluation of the lungs themselves.

CASE 8–2:

MS. G. B.

Ms. G. B. is a 43 year old woman whom you have been caring for since she had resection of a fibrosarcoma of the right thigh 16 months ago. She says that she is well when she comes in for a routine checkup and physical exam is normal. You order routine laboratory studies and a chest x-ray. The radiologist calls you down to see the chest film. What causes her concern?

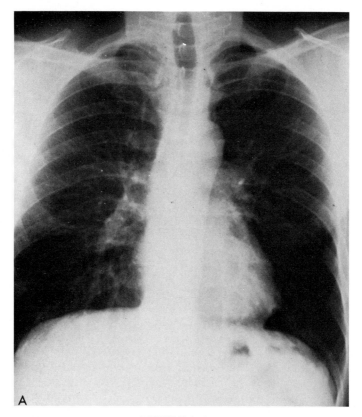

FIGURE 8–2a

There is a 1 cm nodule seen in the lateral aspect of the left midlung that was not seen on older films. No other nodules can be identified. The radiologist suggests that whole lung tomograms be obtained. One film is illustrated.

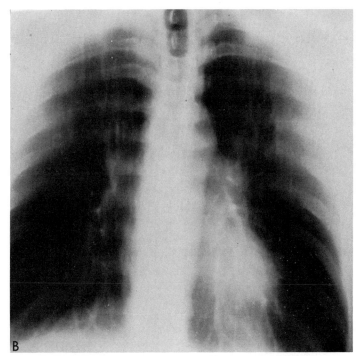

FIGURE 8-2b

The tomograms confirm the presence of a noncalcified nodule in the left lung. No other nodules are seen. The most likely diagnosis is a metastatic deposit. A liver and bone scan are obtained; these show no evidence of other metastatic disease. The oncologist whom you consult suggests that, since there is only a single lesion and the patient is young, the lung lesion should be resected. A thoracic surgeon is called to see the patient and agrees with this plan.

On hearing this, the radiologist suggests that a CT examination of the lungs be performed to exclude other nodules not demonstrated by conventional tomography. The first section shown below was taken just below the carina. The window and mean have been set to demonstrate the soft tissue densities within the lung. Is there any evidence of metastatic disease?

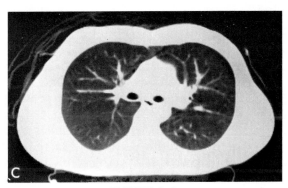

FIGURE 8-2c

This section shows only normal pulmonary vessels. No nodules are seen and the contour of the mediastinum is normal. The low density cleft behind the two mainstem bronchi is air in the esophagus.

The next section is more caudal. What do you observe?

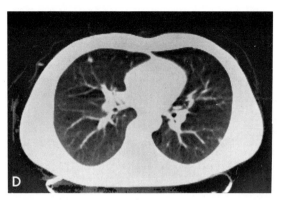

FIGURE 8–2d

There is a well defined nodule in the anterior aspect of the right lung in the anterolateral aspect of the middle lobe. Close scrutiny of the section reveals a second nodule adjacent to the pleura in the posterolateral aspect of the left lower lobe.

What about this section 2 cm more caudal?

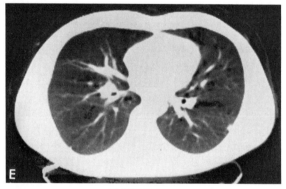

FIGURE 8–2e

Another pleural-based nodule is present in the left lower lobe laterally. A tiny one is seen posteriorly on the right. In further sections several other nodular lesions were discovered.

In view of the patient's history these are believed to be metastases not demonstrated by conventional tomograms. Surgery is cancelled and the patient placed on chemotherapy.

Computerized tomography of the chest can detect nodules not demonstrated by conventional techniques. This is especially true of lesions located in the costophrenic and cardiophrenic recesses and in the subpleural region. The most important use of this technique is in clinical situations in which detection of a single metastasis or additional metastases will significantly alter the patient's management. The major drawback of the technique is that it is not possible to tell whether a particular lesion is benign or malignant. A sizable percentage of lesions discovered by this technique will be benign and of no clinical concern.

One busy afternoon Mr. C. B. drops in without an appointment as is his style. He is a nervous man, inclined to worry about his health, who lives from crisis to crisis. You are chagrined to see him smoking in the waiting area contrary to your advice and that of the conspicuously posted sign. It turns out he has developed some vague chest pain and a morning cough. You are not surprised and remind him about his smoking. He counters that he cannot quit but now is quite concerned that he has cancer. Hoping to reassure him, you send him down the hall for a chest film. What do you see?

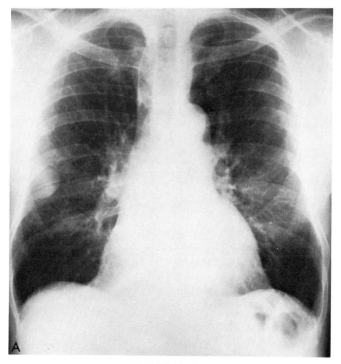

FIGURE 8–3a

There is a sharply defined mass in the right lateral thorax, which is longer than it is deep. The upper and lower margins blend smoothly into the pleural line and do not have acute angles; this suggests an extra-pleural lesion. You think this is probably going to turn out to be benign but Mr. C. B. is positive that he has cancer. When you explain that he must have a biopsy or surgery, he becomes agitated because he believes that this might spread his "cancer." Mr. C. B. asks if anything else might be done and you recall the CT scanner just installed in your building. Thinking this type of examination might add some information, you request the study. Does this prove helpful?

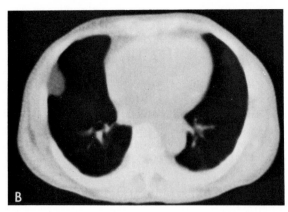

FIGURE 8–3b

The mass has the configuration of an extrapleural lesion. The window and mean have been set to enhance visualization of soft tissues. You should notice that the lesion appears gray while muscle and blood vessels are white. Lung tissue is black. The measured attenuation number within the mass is −93. This is the same as the subcutaneous fat seen in the same section. Is this information helpful?

It is now possible to be confident that this mass represents an extrapleural lipoma, which may be managed without surgery. Mr. C. B. accepts this plan after some discussion. He also says he will try to stop smoking, but you have little hope of this.

Mrs. M. A. is referred to you because of a mass seen at the level of her aortic knob on a routine chest film. She has a strong family history of carcinoma and wants your opinion about her chest films. What do you think?

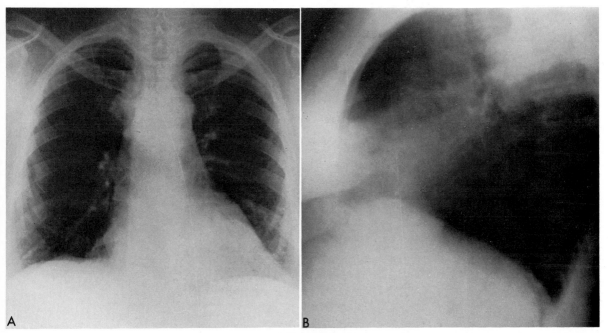

FIGURE 8–4a, b

The mass measures about 4 cm and is seen to the right of the spine just above the carina. Initially, there is concern that this is a carcinoma, but when you compare the current films with others done four and ten years earlier you are sure that the mass, though undetected earlier, is unchanged. You think it may be a cyst, but at 52, Mrs. M. A. is somewhat old for such a lesion. Aneurysm is a consideration but is unlikely because of the location. Its posterior location on the lateral film virtually excludes an aneurysm arising from the ascending aorta and presenting to the right. To exclude a solid mass or unusual aneurysm you decide to do a CT scan before and after infusion of intravenous contrast material. Two scans done before contrast material are illustrated. They were performed 2 cm above the carina and at the level of the carina. What do you see?

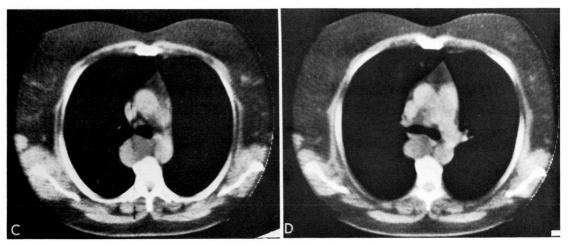

FIGURE 8–4c, d

The descending aorta is seen to the left of the spine, and immediately to the right lies a slightly lower attenuation mass. The cardiac outflow tracts are seen anteriorly in the mediastinum. After contrast material is rapidly infused, repeat studies at similar levels are obtained. What do these demonstrate?

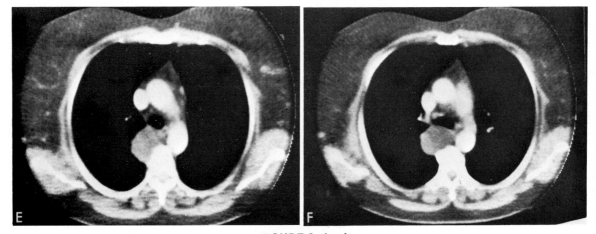

FIGURE 8–4e, f

The mass has remained constant in density and has a low attenuation number, which supports the diagnosis of bronchogenic cyst. The great vessels are densely opacified on this study; therefore, an aneurysm with a patent lumen can be excluded. Clotted aneurysms and solid tumors for the most part will have a greater attenuation than is seen here. Mrs. M. A. is satisfied and no surgery is performed. Two years later, there is still no change in her chest film.

MISS L. B.

Miss L. B., a student nurse, has been working on the pulmonary unit. When she comes in complaining of malaise, night sweats and a lump in her neck, you are inclined to dismiss her complaints as those of a suggestable young woman. On physical examination, however, there are some enlarged, firm left cervical nodes. A chest film increases your concern and a biopsy shows histiocytic lymphoma. Her preoperative chest radiograph is shown below. What do you see?

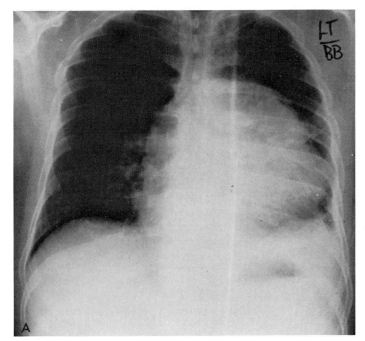

FIGURE 8–5a

There is a large mediastinal mass and a left pleural effusion. The descending aorta and aortic knob are not seen. The left mainstem bronchus seems displaced downward.

Clearly, this unfortunate young woman has extensive lymphoma. Before decisions about therapy are made, studies are obtained to better evaluate the extent of disease. Since a CT evaluation of the abdomen is requested, sections of the chest are also obtained to aid in radiation port planning. A single section at the level of the carina is illustrated. What is seen?

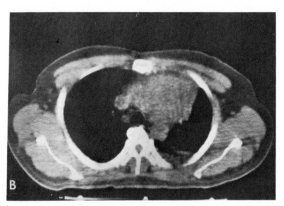

FIGURE 8–5b

There is a large mediastinal mass extending into the left hemi-thorax. The superior vena cava is seen on the right lateral margin of the mediastinum. Adjacent to this is the ascending aorta, which cannot be separated from the mass. The pulmonary outflow tract can be identified. The descending aorta is seen to the left of the spine but its anterior margin is obliterated. Pleural fluid and compressed lung are seen in the left posterior hemithorax.

This extensive lymphomatous mass has infiltrated the mediastinum, obliterating normal fat planes. While no surgery was planned in this case, these are findings that indicate nonresectability for cure in a mediastinal mass. Position of the great vessels would be better seen after a bolus injection of contrast material.

Mrs. T. S. comes to your office complaining of chest pain and non-productive cough. She has always been in good health and does not smoke but has been bothered by chest pain and some weakness for the last several months. A routine chest film is requested and brings a surprising result. What is your opinion?

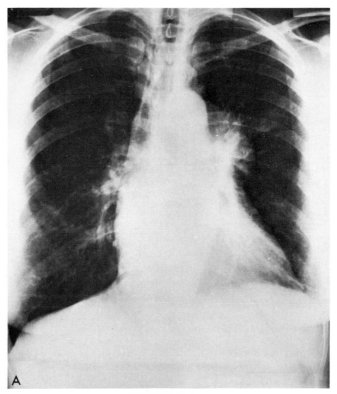

FIGURE 8–6a

A large mass is superimposed on the left hilum. Pulmonary vessels are seen through the mass and the descending aorta is normal, indicating an anterior location. No rim of calcification is seen to suggest an aneurysm. The mass is not clearly mediastinal. A CT scan is ordered to better define the nature, location and extent of the lesion. The first section is above the level of the aortic arch. A bolus injection of intravenous contrast material has been given to opacify the vessels. What information is obtained?

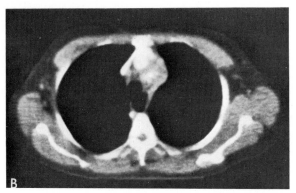

FIGURE 8–6b

Air is seen in the trachea and esophagus and there is intense opacification of the great vessels. There is a bulge in the contour of the left superior mediastinum. The section at the level of the aortic arch shows the abnormality to greater advantage. What do you see?

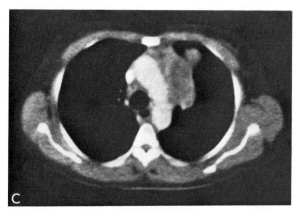

FIGURE 8–6c

The superior vena cava on the right and the aortic arch are intensely opacified. There is a large left mediastinal mass, which has a mottled consistency. The mass is not separated from the aortic arch by normal mediastinal fat and extends into the adjacent lung. The next section is below the aortic arch. What do you see?

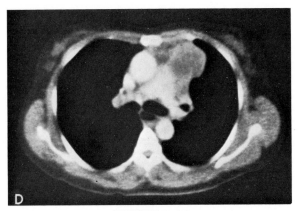

FIGURE 8–6d

The large mass is separated from the anterior chest wall by a fat plane, but its posterior aspect is not separable from the main pulmonary artery and the left hilum.

The pattern here is that of an extensive infiltrating mediastinal mass, which would not be completely resectable. At surgery, the lesion is found to be an infiltrating malignant thymoma that the surgeon could only biopsy. Mrs. T. S. has a good initial response to radiation.

CT OF SOFT TISSUES AND SKELETON

Radiographic evaluation of soft tissue detail is dependent on the ability to discriminate very small differences in tissue x-ray attenuation. The remarkable sensitivity of CT to differences in soft tissue x-ray attenuation, compared to that of conventional radiographic techniques, gives CT a significant place in the examination of the soft tissues of the body wall and extremities. The cross sectional scans display the various tissue planes well. It is generally easy to determine the relationship of a pathological process to the muscle, fascia and fat of the body wall and to the muscle bundles of the extremities.

In the examination of the bones, CT provides a transaxial view that cannot be obtained by conventional radiographic methods. Specific relationships that are difficult to judge on conventional views are easily determined.

There is a clear separation of the medullary canal of bone, the cortex and the surrounding soft tissues. The internal structure of bone lesions can be assessed and the extent of a lesion within the bone can be seen. Replacement of the marrow in the medullary space may be seen as a change in its normal fat density.

The bilateral symmetry of the human body facilitates comparison of the normal structures on one side of the body with the abnormal extremity or side. It is wise to remember that past trauma, neurological disorders or developmental abnormalities may cause asymmetry that can be confusing though not of immediate clinical concern. Therefore, though side to side comparison is generally useful, it must be done with knowledge of the individual patient.

CT has a unique capability in evaluation of soft tissue abnormalities. It should be stressed that the need for this particular capability will not be frequent. Certainly, most soft tissue lesions do not need CT scanning. CT should be reserved for situations in which it will really add useful information.

MRS. R. P. AND MR. S. B.

Mrs. R. P. is an extremely obese 68 year old woman who has returned to see you because of a lump near her mastectomy scar. The lump is firm and you suspect she has a recurrence of her breast carcinoma. Your physical examination is somewhat impeded by Mrs. R. P.'s obesity, but you think there is another mass in the right lateral abdominal wall. Fearing a second metastasis, you order a CT scan to confirm your physical finding.

A single section through the mass is shown. What do you see?

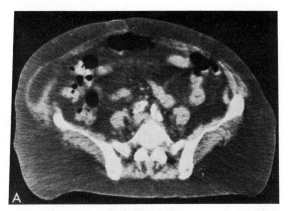

FIGURE 9–1a

The layers of oblique abdominal wall muscles are separated by an ovoid mass. Most important, its attenuation is the same as the surrounding adipose tissue, indicating that the mass is composed of fatty tissue and is not a metastasis. Incidentally, there is marked calcification of both common iliac arteries.

No other metastases are turned up. Mrs. R. P. does well with local radiation therapy to the single area of recurrence near her mastectomy scar.

Mr. S. B. is a 78 year old man who comes to see you because of swelling of his right thigh. He says the swelling has been present for about six weeks, but because he seems a bit confused you think this may be inaccurate. The right thigh is about twice the size of the left at physical examination. It has a slightly soft, doughy consistency and is not tender or inflamed. Films are taken of the thigh. What do you see?

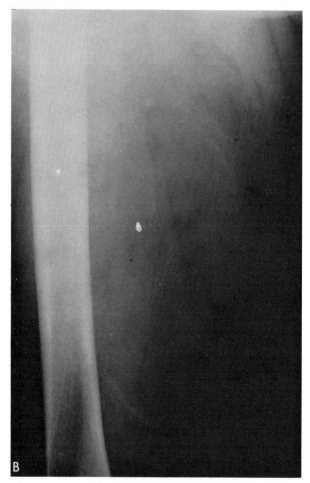

FIGURE 9–1b

There is a poorly defined large fat density mass medial to the femur. It appears to be partially encapsulated. You are rather sure that Mr. S. B. has a lipoma, but the six week history is worrisome. Lipomas grow slowly, whereas liposarcomas can be much more aggressive. CT scan is ordered to try to make this differentiation and to define the relationship of the tumor to the major vessels and muscles of the thigh. Two sections taken through the mass are shown. What do they show?

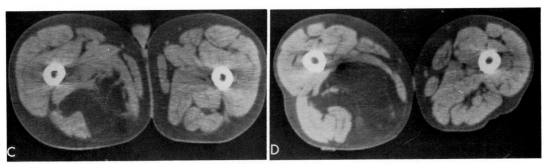

FIGURE 9–1c, d

The left thigh is a normal control, and the relationships of the various muscle bellies, vessels and surrounding fat and connective tissue are well shown. The saphenous vein is seen in the subcutaneous fat medially. The superficial femoral artery is hard to identify but the deep femoral artery and vein are well seen, especially on the lower section. All the major muscle groups are seen, including among others the vastus group, the strap muscles and the biceps femoris. On the right the tumor is fatty, and though it spreads and distorts muscles, it does not seem to invade any of the muscles. The deep vascular pedicle is also engulfed. Both the absence of invasion and the pure fatty appearance make lipoma more likely as a diagnosis than liposarcoma, which is more cellular.

Surgery is performed and a yellow fatty tumor is easily removed. Microscopic sections reveal a benign lipoma. While most lipomas need no radiologic evaluation, these cases demonstrate the value of CT scanning in selected cases.

CASE 9–2:

MRS. Q. T.

Mrs. Q. T. is an unfortunate woman who is referred for a CT scan to help plan radiation therapy ports. Five years ago, she had a left radical mastectomy for carcinoma. She did well for three years; then a mass that was felt in the right breast also proved to be malignant. A right radical mastectomy was performed and radiation therapy was given. Now she has a firm mass palpable just below the right clavicle. What do you make of this CT section?

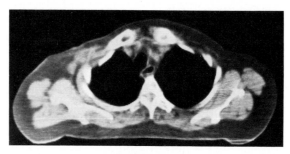

FIGURE 9–2

This section was done through the upper chest at the level of the palpable mass. The scapulae, medial portions of the clavicles and the muscles of the shoulder girdle are well seen. Air is present in the esophagus, which is immediately anterior to the vertebral body. The trachea is ventral and to the right of the esophagus.

Examination of the soft tissues of the anterior chest wall show both sides to be abnormal, since the pectoral muscles have been removed during the bilateral radical mastectomies. On the left, there is normal subcutaneous fat over the anterior chest wall. On the right, the subcutaneous fat has been partially replaced by a lobular mass extending toward the axilla. The mass has an attenuation similar to muscle and is recurrence of breast carcinoma in the chest wall.

Additional sections were performed both above and below this section so that the total volume of tumor recurrence could be determined and the proper radiation therapy port planned.

Mr. T. K. is a 45 year old man who had an extensive retroperitoneal liposarcoma resected eight months ago. Now he feels a lump in his right side, which is growing slowly. The examining surgeon finds a mass near the inferior aspect of Mr. T. K.'s incision that he believes to be an intra-abdominal tumor recurrence. Prior to surgery a CT scan is requested to better define the mass. Where do you think the location of the mass is?

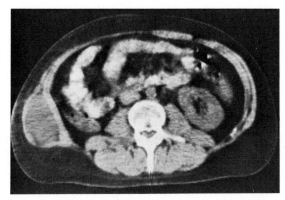

FIGURE 9–3

The scan demonstrates an ovoid mass, which is totally confined to the right abdominal wall, lying between the external oblique and the internal oblique muscles. Obviously the mass is not within the abdominal cavity or retroperitoneum. Did you notice anything else about the abdominal musculature?

When you compare the musculature on the right with that of the left, it is apparent that the anterior aspects of the muscles on the right abdominal wall and the right rectus muscle are atrophied. This was probably caused by the recent surgical incision. What do you make of the density of the mass itself?

The mass is less dense than the surrounding muscles but more dense than the normal retroperitoneal fat, and the internal character of the mass is quite homogeneous. While it is difficult to be specific about histologic diagnosis on the basis of attenuation values, the findings and the history strongly suggest a recurrence of liposarcoma.

Since the remainder of the examination is unremarkable, the recurrence of the liposarcoma probably represents a surgical implant in the abdominal wall rather than extension of the original tumor. The implant is excised and Mr. T. K. does well for some months.

MR. W. R.

Mr. W. R. is a 34 year old man whom you have been following closely since you removed a small malignant melanoma from his back about 18 months ago. He has felt well during this interval but begins to complain of a full sensation on movement of his left shoulder. While you are sure he has a recurrence of his melanoma, physical examination and left shoulder x-rays are normal. A followup visit is scheduled for eight weeks, but the patient shows up earlier with an obvious mass in his left axilla. Biopsy confirms a recurrence and palliative therapy is planned. One consideration is excision. A CT scan is ordered to assess the full extent of the mass.

Three sections, one just below the axilla, one through the lower chest and one at about L2, are shown. What do you see on the first scan?

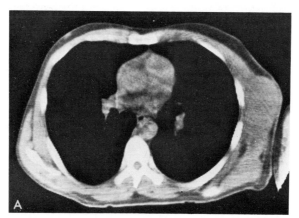

FIGURE 9–4a

This section demonstrates the bulky soft tissue mass in the left axilla. Use the opposite side for comparison. The window settings have been adjusted for thoracic wall soft tissues and lung detail is obscured. Is more information available on the next section?

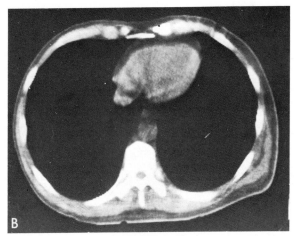

FIGURE 9–4b

The asymmetry of the chest wall soft tissues is still quite apparent on this scan, though palpation at this level is equivocal for a mass. You are certain no mass is felt below this level.

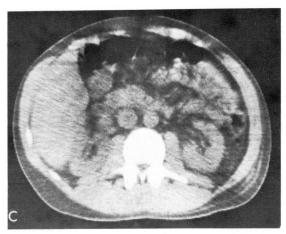

FIGURE 9–4c

The third section, at the level of the L2 vertebral body, reveals a fine tongue of tumor still present about 8 cm caudad of any palpable mass. The intraabdominal contents are normal. The extent of the bulky and sheet-like tumor is so great that surgery is not considered feasible. Chemotherapy gives some initial relief.

The CT scan is uniquely able to detect soft tissue abnormalities of this nature. No previous diagnostic method could have demonstrated tumor extension beyond the obvious palpable mass.

MRS. V. P.

Mrs. V. P. had surgery for an ovarian carcinoma about ten years ago. Some positive nodes were found in the specimen and she had radiation therapy in the hope of providing a cure. She developed a radiation cystitis after the therapy but has handled the discomfort well and has remained free of clinical tumor recurrence.

You are therefore dismayed when she comes to your office complaining of marked tenderness over the pubic symphysis. You find that she has extreme tenderness, especially to the left of the midline and, in addition, there is some questionable fullness. Tumor recurrence with bony involvement is your primary concern, but films of the pelvis are normal. Because of the radiation cystitis, Mrs. V. P.'s bladder cannot be distended enough to get a good pelvic ultrasound, but the ultrasonographer comments that her soft tissues do not transmit sound normally. He also suggests a pelvic CT scan as an alternative technique for visualization of the pelvis.

Mrs. V. P. has developed a spiking fever and her tenderness has increased. You request a pelvic CT scan, which is performed after the intravenous and oral contrast medium have been given. Three sections from the examination are illustrated. What are the pertinent observations on the first scan?

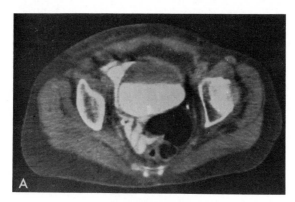

FIGURE 9–5a

This section is made about 6 cm cephalad of the symphysis pubis. The bladder is filled with urine and there is a sharp fluid level between opacified and nonopacified urine. Small bowel loops are seen to the right of the bladder. The distal sigmoid colon and rectum are gas filled. Both ureters are opacified with contrast medium. The left is easy to identify, while the right is somewhat obscured by the small bowel loops. The important observation on this section is a negative one. No masses or increased soft tissues are present that might suggest tumor recurrence. How about the next section?

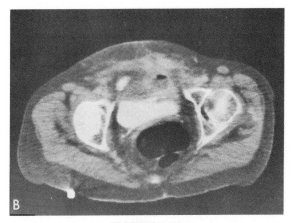

FIGURE 9–5b

The second section, about 3 cm lower, again demonstrates colon and bladder, but anterior to the contrast-filled bladder on the left is a poorly defined soft tissue mass with an air-fluid level. No bowel should be in this location and there is no continuity of this mass with other bowel to suggest an unusual hernia. An abscess is the lesion most likely to have this appearance. Is there more useful information on the next scan?

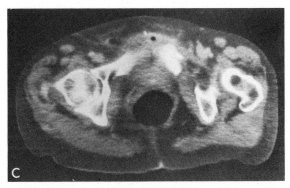

FIGURE 9–5c

This section is at the very top of the symphysis pubis. Again a small pocket of air is seen in the anterior abdominal wall. All the bones seen are normal and no other soft tissue abnormalities are seen.

The diagnosis is an abscess in the soft tissues of the anterior abdominal wall. Carefully coned-down radiographs of the area demonstrate pockets of air (arrow).

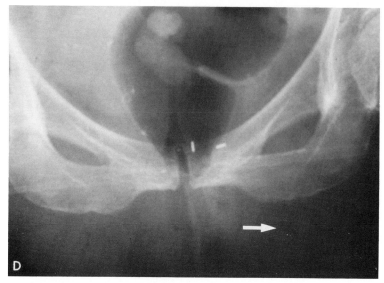

FIGURE 9–5d

At surgery more than 300 ml of purulent material is evacuated from the abscess. No cause of the abscess is found but the patient's recovery is uneventful.

Mr. B. W. is a troublesome 24 year old who abuses multiple drugs, both orally and by injection. Now he has been hospitalized with right sacroiliac pain and you suspect that he is trying to obtain pain medication. He complains constantly and seems to have some tenderness. What do the radiographs of the area show?

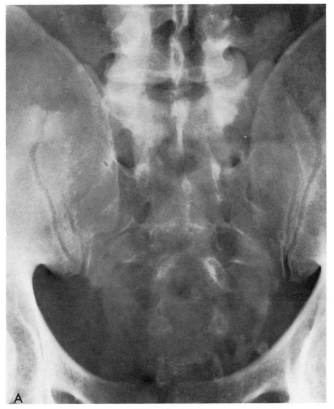

FIGURE 9–6a

There is an area of increased bony density that seems to extend across the right sacroiliac joint; it could be due to an indolent joint infection. A radionuclide bone scan is also positive in this area. Conventional tomograms are then requested. What do you think?

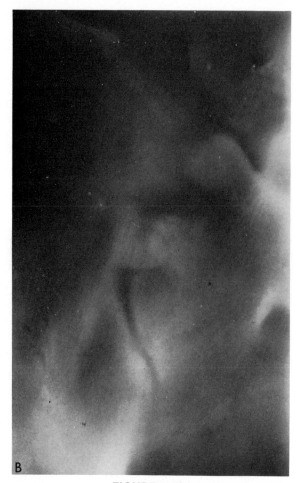

FIGURE 9–6b

The bony sclerosis seems to bridge the joint and suggests osteophytes. A CT scan is ordered to evaluate the lesion. The section is made through the abnormal area and the window and mean have been set to demonstrate bone detail. What is shown?

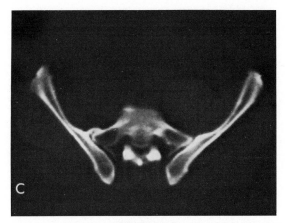

FIGURE 9–6c

This section clearly shows bridging of the right sacroiliac joint by a degenerative spur without any evidence of bony destruction. These changes are seen to good advantage in the transaxial view because of the orientation of the sacroiliac joint. Further investigation is not warranted and the patient is discharged to a drug rehabilitation program.

CASE 9–7:

MISS D. O.

Miss D. O. complains of pain in her low back on the right side. You would like to ignore her complaints, but she is your office receptionist and knows how useful x-rays are. Rather than hear her complain daily, you decide to prove that nothing is wrong and order films of the lumbar spine and pelvis. What do you see in the pelvis?

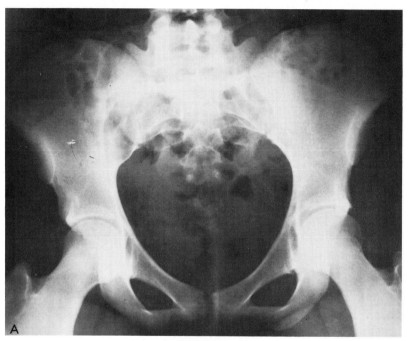

FIGURE 9–7a

Much to your surprise, there is an ovoid lucency adjacent to the right sacroiliac joint. This is very sharply marginated and has a benign appearance. Miss D. O. is excited about this discovery and you refer her to an orthopedic surgeon. He orders a bone scan. What do you see?

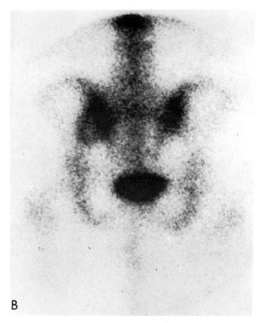

FIGURE 9-7b

The lesion in the iliac bone adjacent to the sacroiliac joint is seen as a rim of radionuclide uptake with a central void. The findings are most compatible with a benign lesion such as a bone cyst or fibrous lesion. An indolent infection is also a consideration. Prior to exploration, a CT scan is suggested to evaluate the nature and location of the lesion. What do you see?

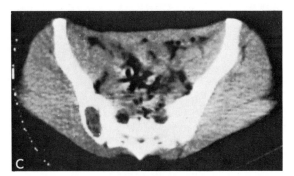

FIGURE 9-7c

The lesion is again seen in the posterior aspect of the iliac bone just lateral to the sacroiliac joint. It is very sharply defined and the contents are less dense than adjacent muscle. The measured attenuation is +3, very close to that of water. This makes a bone cyst the most likely diagnosis.

The surgeon is very happy about the localization obtained and a posterior approach is planned. At surgery, a bone cyst is found and treated with curettement and packing with bone chips. Miss D. O. recovers rapidly and returns to work, delighted with her own clinical acumen.

CASE 9–8:

MR. J. Q.

Mr. J. Q. is a 17 year old high school football player who complains that his left thigh has been painful for a month, especially while playing. He thinks he injured himself during a workout but is worried because the injury doesn't seem to be getting better. Physical examination reveals limitation of motion. There are also several furuncles on his torso, which he says are common for him. You order radiographs of the hip. There is a striking finding. What is it?

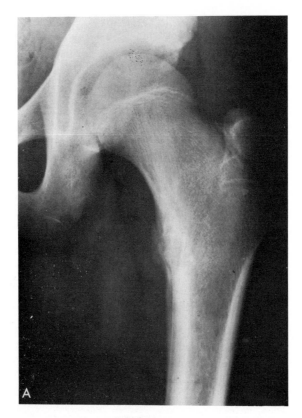

FIGURE 9–8a

There is an area of bony destruction that is probably associated with the lesser trochanter. There is also lamellated periosteal new bone. You think that this may be a chronic osteomyelitis and call in an orthopedic surgeon, who requests tomograms. Do these add any information?

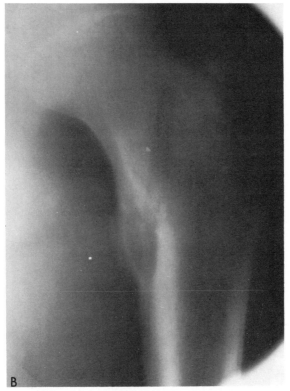

FIGURE 9–8b

These confirm the presence of a lesion that is compatible with your clinical diagnosis but little further information is gained. The surgeon plans to explore the thigh; it would help him to know where the lesion really is. A CT scan is requested to locate and evaluate the lesion. A single section is shown. What do you think? Use the normal right side for comparison.

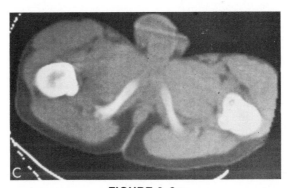

FIGURE 9–8c

It is clear that the abnormality does not involve the lesser trochanter but is in the anteromedial femoral cortex. The lesion has a dense rim of new bone. A sequestrum can be seen with certainty by adjusting the mean and window settings. The change in localization alters the surgical approach and the surgeon is happy with the information. At surgery, chronic osteomyelitis is encountered. This responds to drainage and antibiotics and Mr. J. Q. is able to return rapidly to the gridiron.

CASE 9–9:

MR. M. C.

Mr. M. C., a 25 year old graduate student, is admitted to the hospital for abdominal pain. This is due to gastroenteritis but, on the admitting physical examination, a painless mass is noted adjacent to the upper aspect of the left tibia. The patient says this has been present for about two years. What do you think of the radiograph?

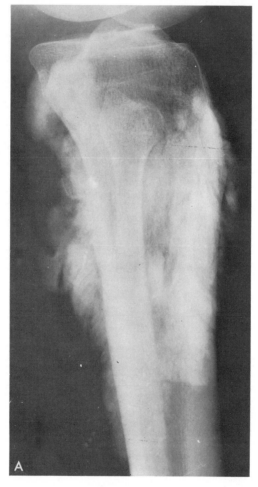

FIGURE 9–9a

There is a large ossified soft tissue mass that surrounds the upper tibia. Tomography is obtained. What are your impressions?

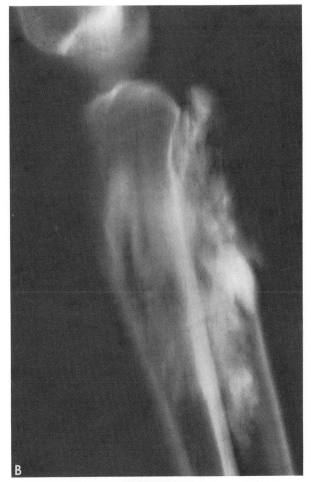

FIGURE 9–9b

The lobulated ossified mass extends posteriorly. Inferiorly, there is a thin lucency that separates the mass from the posterior cortex of the tibia. These findings strongly suggest a parosteal type of osteosarcoma. However, increased density is present in the medullary canal. This may be artifactual, but it is important to be sure, since extensive intramedullary tumor suggests the more usual osteogenic sarcoma, a lesion with a much different prognosis. You decide to examine the lesion by CT scan. The first section is through the lower aspect of the mass.

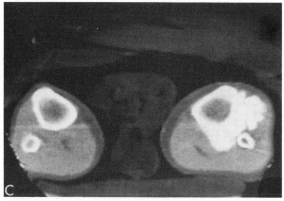

FIGURE 9–9c

The mass is seen at the posterolateral aspect of the tibia. Laterally, there is a thin separation of the mass from the bone itself. The next section is through the midportion of the mass. What do you see?

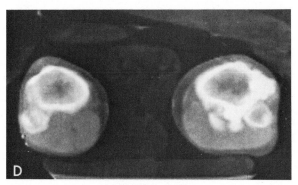

FIGURE 9–9d

Here the ossified mass surrounds the lateral and posterior portions of the tibia. There is a broadbased attachment. The tibial medullary cavity is slightly encroached upon. The fibula is normal. The next section is higher, through the upper aspect of the mass. What is seen here?

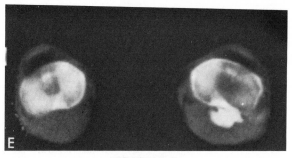

FIGURE 9–9e

Here some more encroachment of the bone tumor can be seen on the medullary space of the tibia, but this seems to extend in from the mass. This appearance is most compatible with parosteal osteosarcoma. Heterotopic ossification such as myositis ossificans is excluded, and an osteogenic sarcoma is highly unlikely, since they grow from the inside out. The patient is treated with wide resection and bone grafting. The pathological specimen is identified as parosteal osteosarcoma.

INDEX